HIV/AIDS: A Very Short Introduction

VERY SHORT INTRODUCTIONS are for anyone wanting a stimulating and accessible way in to a new subject. They are written by experts, and have been published in more than 25 languages worldwide.

The series began in 1995, and now represents a wide variety of topics in history, philosophy, religion, science, and the humanities. The VSI Library now contains over 200 volumes—a Very Short Introduction to everything from ancient Egypt and Indian philosophy to conceptual art and cosmology—and will continue to grow to a library of around 300 titles.

Very Short Introductions available now:

For more information visit our web site:
www.oup.co.uk/general/vsi/

Alan Whiteside

HIV/AIDS

A Very Short Introduction

OXFORD
UNIVERSITY PRESS

OXFORD
UNIVERSITY PRESS

Great Clarendon Street, Oxford OX2 6DP

Oxford University Press is a department of the University of Oxford.
It furthers the University's objective of excellence in research, scholarship,
and education by publishing worldwide in

Oxford New York

Auckland Cape Town Dar es Salaam Hong Kong Karachi
Kuala Lumpur Madrid Melbourne Mexico City Nairobi
New Delhi Shanghai Taipei Toronto

With offices in

Argentina Austria Brazil Chile Czech Republic France Greece
Guatemala Hungary Italy Japan Poland Portugal Singapore
South Korea Switzerland Thailand Turkey Ukraine Vietnam

Oxford is a registered trade mark of Oxford University Press
in the UK and in certain other countries

Published in the United States
by Oxford University Press Inc., New York

British Library Cataloguing in Publication Data

Data available

Library of Congress Cataloging in Publication Data

Data available

ISBN 978-0-19-280692-5

7 9 10 8

Typeset by SPI Publisher Services, Pondicherry, India
Printed in Great Britain by
Ashford Colour Press Ltd, Gosport, Hampshire

Contents

Preface

It is over a quarter of a century since clinicians in the USA identified the first cases of the syndrome that came to be known as AIDS. These reports simply referred to groups of people with unusual illnesses. Today AIDS is the major killer of young adults, globally 40 million people are infected, the vast majority in developing countries, and numbers continue to rise.

I first took notice of HIV/AIDS in 1987 when researching labour migration in Southern Africa. Apartheid and the legacy of colonialism created the perfect hothouse for the spread of a sexually transmitted disease. What started as an academic and intellectual exercise became intensely personal. The HIV prevalence in Swaziland, where I grew up, rose from 3.9% among pregnant women in 1992, to 42.6% in the 2004 survey. I live in South Africa, where AIDS affects us all as we watch colleagues, friends, neighbours, and co-workers fall ill and die. We converse about and take these deaths in our stride in a way that is abnormal but unremarked.

We have made huge progress in understanding the science of the retrovirus that causes AIDS: where it came from, how it works, and how it spreads; we are still a long way from having a cure or vaccine and have proven lamentably inadequate at stopping its progress in many communities. Medical advances mean that there are treatments available that can prolong life, although they are expensive and complex and do not cure.

This Very Short Introduction is about a unique and dynamic disease that has long-term consequences. It provides an introduction to the science around the pandemic but focuses on the profound impacts AIDS is having on households, communities, and on national demographic and development indicators. We are seeing adults dying, orphans left behind, women unevenly burdened by care, impacts on civil society groups, on politicians, and a general atmosphere of 'dis-ease'. In order to understand the effects of AIDS, we need to extend the time frame, to take a longer-term perspective: macro impacts take decades to unfold. This disease is a long-wave event, and we must look into the future to understand and respond to its consequences.

The burden of HIV/AIDS is not borne equally. It is the deprived and powerless who are most likely to be infected and affected. AIDS is primarily a disease of the poor, be they poor nations or poor people in rich nations. Geographically the worst epidemics are in sub-Saharan Africa, specifically Southern Africa, and many examples in this introduction are drawn from here.

HIV/AIDS is a global phenomenon but the dynamics and its consequences are played out differently across the world. This introduction looks at the epidemics and what they mean for countries, populations, production, and reproduction. It reflects that AIDS calls on us to assess what is important to us and how we relate to each other, in our communities but also globally. It asks if it matters if a young Swazi girl has a greater than 80% chance of dying from AIDS in her lifetime. What does it mean for older women caring for their children's children? The answers are not clear or simple. There are unexpected signs of hope. In particular, there is a coming together in South African society that is reminiscent of the fight against apartheid. Will this mobilization and unity so essential to stopping the disease be repeated elsewhere?

Writing a short book proved more difficult than I would ever have believed. I would like to express my appreciation to many people for their help and support: the OUP staff, in particular Luciana O'Flaherty, who read and commented on numerous drafts, Marsha Filion, and James Thompson; in Durban, the Health Economics and HIV/AIDS Research Division staff; my family Ailsa Marcham, Rowan Whiteside, and Douglas Whiteside; and friends, colleagues, and readers, specifically Tony Barnett, May Chazan, Stephanie Nixon, Nana Poku, Judith Shier, Tim Quinlan, Obed Qulo, Jon Simon, and Alex de Waal, and the OUP readers.

Abbreviations

AIDS	acquired immunodeficiency syndrome
ANC	antenatal clinic
ART	antiretroviral therapies
AZT	azidothymidine
CBR	crude birth rate
CDR	crude death rate
CDC	Centers for Disease Control
CIHD	Center for International Health and Development
DFID	Department for International Development
DNA	deoxyribonucleic acid
DHS	demographic health survey
ELISA	enzyme-linked immunosorbent assay
GDP	gross domestic product
GPA	Global Programme on AIDS
HDI	Human Development Index
HIV	human immunodeficiency virus
IDU	intravenous drug user
MDG	Millennium Development Goal
MDR TB	multi-drug-resistant tuberculosis
MTCT	mother-to-child transmission
NGO	non-governmental organization
PEPFAR	Presidential Emergency Plan for AIDS Relief
RNA	ribonucleic acid
SARS	severe acute respiratory syndrome
SIDA	*syndrome d'immunodéficience acquise*
SIV	simian immunodeficiency viruses
SSA	sub-Saharan Africa
STI	sexually transmitted infection

TAC	Treatment Action Campaign
TB	tuberculosis
TFR	total fertility rate
UNAIDS	Joint United Nations Programme on HIV/AIDS
UNDP	United Nations Development Programme
UNFPA	United Nations Fund for Population Activities
UNICEF	United Nations Children's Fund
USAID	United States Agency for International Development
WHO	World Health Organization
XDR TB	extensively drug-resistant tuberculosis

List of illustrations

The publisher and the author apologize for any errors or omissions in the above list. If contacted they will be pleased to rectify these at the earliest opportunity.

List of tables

Chapter 1
The emergence and state of the HIV/AIDS epidemic

The identification of HIV/AIDS

Acquired immunodeficiency syndrome (AIDS) is caused by the human immunodeficiency virus (HIV), which crossed from primates into humans. Although isolated cases of infection in people may have appeared earlier, the first cases of the current epidemic probably occurred in the 1930s, and the disease spread rapidly in the 1970s.

AIDS was publicly reported on 5 June 1981, in the Morbidity and Mortality Weekly Report produced by the Centers for Disease Control (CDC) in Atlanta in the USA. Doctors recorded unexpected clusters of previously extremely rare diseases such as *Pneumocystis carinii*, a type of pneumonia, and Kaposi's sarcoma, a normally slow-growing tumour. These conditions manifested in exceptionally serious forms, and in a narrowly defined risk group – young homosexual men.

It soon became apparent that these illnesses were occurring in other definable groups: haemophiliacs, blood transfusion recipients, and intravenous drug users (IDUs). By 1982, cases were being seen among the partners and infants of those infected. The name: acquired immunodeficiency syndrome, acronym AIDS, was agreed in Washington in July 1982. In the same year the CDC produced a working definition for AIDS based on clinical signs. AIDS describes the disease accurately: people acquire the condition; it results in a deficiency within the immune system; and it is a syndrome not a single disease. In French, Portuguese, and Spanish, it is known as SIDA, the full French name being *syndrome d'immunodéficience acquise.*

Beyond North America, there was news of cases from Europe, Australia, New Zealand, Latin America, especially Brazil and Mexico, and Africa. In Zambia, a significant rise in cases of Kaposi's sarcoma was recorded. In Kinshasa in the Democratic Republic of the Congo, there was an upsurge in patients with cryptococcosis, an unusual fungal infection. The Ugandan Ministry of Health was receiving reports of increased and unexpected deaths in Lake Victoria fishing villages.

Even when the syndrome had been identified and named, it was not clear what its cause was, how it spread, or which treatments were effective or could be developed. Scientists agreed the most likely origin was a, then unidentified, virus. The hunt for this was intense in laboratories across the world, with international collaboration, and sharing of specimens and tissue. In 1983 the virus was identified by the Institut Pasteur in France, which called it Lymphadenopathy-Associated Virus, or LAV. In April 1984 in the US, the National Cancer Institute (NCI) isolated the virus and named it HTLV-III. There was an unseemly spat when the US Secretary for Health and Human Services announced to the world that the NCI was responsible for the scientific breakthrough that identified HIV. The face-saving compromise was to say French and US laboratories had both identified the cause of AIDS. In 1987 the name 'human immunodeficiency virus' was confirmed by the International Committee on Taxonomy of Viruses.

Many diseases spread from animals to humans (and the other way). These are called zoonoses. Recent examples include severe acute respiratory syndrome (SARS), which was tracked to civet cats, and avian influenza (bird flu). HIV is, so far, the most deadly pathogen to have made this leap: Ebola virus is more infectious but can be contained; SARS, fortunately, was not as infectious; avian flu has not yet taken hold in humans, but is cause for concern.

Initially there was a degree of hysteria around AIDS, where it came from, and how it was transmitted. In San Francisco, when it was identified as a gay men's disease, police and fire officers feared they would be infected through exposure to blood and body fluids from homosexuals. In 1983 officers were given face masks and gloves and educated on how to protect themselves from this alleged risk. Today, when AIDS hits the headlines in the West, which is not often, most stories fall into a few categories: what the West (and Western celebrities) are doing to assist the worst affected countries and communities, such as supporting orphanages and adopting orphans; the impoverishment and misery AIDS causes; the continued spread among certain groups – IDUs in the former Soviet countries or Chinese peasants; and, in rich countries, the deliberate spreading of the virus by individuals to implicitly 'innocent victims'.

Having identified how HIV was spread, the challenge was to reduce transmission. Early responses were technical: improving blood safety, providing condoms, and encouraging safe injecting practices. Soon it became apparent that these were not enough, behaviours needed to change. At the same time, the race was on to find drugs that could cure or, at least, treat infected people. It took 15 years to develop effective antiretroviral therapies (ART), and this advance was announced at the 1996 International AIDS Conference in Vancouver.

There is still little understanding of the long-term impact of the epidemic. While the worst predictions of national collapse, rising levels of crime, economic stagnation, and general malaise won't come about, vulnerabilities, like the epidemic, will be differentiated. The poorest bear the burden.

The long-wave epidemic

AIDS is new: in 2006, the 25th anniversary of its identification, there were close to 40 million people around the world living with HIV and over 20 million had died. Globally the number of infections had increased rapidly. This growth has slowed but continues steadily, however it is confined to specific locations; the feared uncontrollable worldwide pandemic has not occurred.

The virus itself is unusual, as explained in detail in the next chapter. The most common mode of transmission is sexual intercourse, followed by mother-to-child infection, sharing drug-injecting equipment, and contaminated blood or instruments in health care settings. Because transmission is mainly through sex or drug use and there is no cure, there is much prejudice and fear. HIV/AIDS was and remains stigmatizing at an individual and national level.

HIV/AIDS is a complex long-wave event: there are waves of spread and waves of impact. This concept is illustrated by the three curves shown in Figure 1. The first shows the prevalence rising steadily and levelling off, a silent spread. The second curve, six to ten years later, is the cumulative number of AIDS cases. These are visible but diffused across a nation, and each year the numbers are small. Those studying HIV know infections will develop into illnesses and, untreated, lead to death. At T_1 the number of cases at T_2 can be predicted and should be planned for. The third curve, even further in the future, is the impact, which is harder to predict and plan for.

Some idea of the timescale comes from Uganda. Here HIV prevalence peaked in about 1989, and the number of AIDS

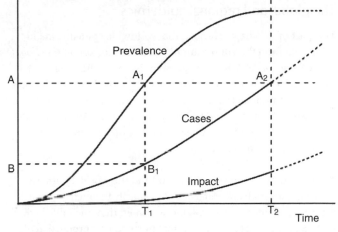

1. Epidemic curves

orphans peaked 14 years later in 2003. In countries such as South Africa, where HIV prevalence may not have peaked, the number of orphans could still be rising in 2020. Orphaned children carry the effects of being orphaned for the rest of their lives. Impacts last for generations. The diagram shows three of the waves; there will be others and the impact will be long term.

The future of HIV/AIDS is, epidemiologically speaking, reasonably predictable. Unless the virus mutates and becomes more easily transmitted, it will be contained. Science is advancing and new treatments are becoming available. Technological prevention methods, such as microbicides and vaccines, are being developed, although these are still some years away.

The impacts are less certain, but will be confined to the worst affected regions, notably parts of Africa; and most marginal groups. Due to the specific demographics of declining and ageing populations, some Eastern European countries may be particularly adversely impacted.

The global and regional epidemics

This part of the chapter reviews the worldwide epidemic mainly using data from the 2006 biannual UNAIDS *Report on the Global AIDS Epidemic*. HIV has not spread uniformly. Although most early reported cases were among gay men in the USA and Europe, the greatest numbers have consistently been African. In 1980 there were about 18,000 HIV infections in North America, 1,000 each in Europe and Latin America, and 41,000 in sub-Saharan Africa. Table 1 shows current data.

There are different sub-epidemics around the world. Southern Africa has an epidemic transmitted primarily through heterosexual intercourse, with more women than men infected. In Asia total numbers are alarming but small as a proportion of the populations. The East European and central Asian epidemics have been principally fuelled by IDUs and are growing. In rich countries the epidemic is contained, and mainly seen among marginal groups, although numbers are slowly rising.

Sub-Saharan Africa has the largest number of people living with HIV: two-thirds (64%) of infected people and three-quarters of all infected women live here. There are differences in the sizes and trajectories of African epidemics. Southern Africa has the worst epidemic, with the numbers infected still rising in some countries. South Africa's antenatal clinic survey recorded an increased prevalence from 29.5% in 2004 to 30.2% in 2005, but this fell to 29.1% in 2006, and there are other hopeful signs: data from Zimbabwe and Zambia also suggest a fall in prevalence. In Zimbabwe, HIV prevalence in pregnant women fell from 26% in 2002 to 21% in 2004, and in younger women (15–24) the drop was from 29% to 20% between 2000 and 2004.

In most of West Africa, HIV seems not to have spread. Senegal is held as a model for successful prevention: HIV prevalence was below 1% throughout the 1980s and 1990s, increasing slightly to

Table 1. Regional HIV and AIDS statistics, 2003 and 2005

Country	Adults (15+) and children living with HIV	Adults (15+) and children newly infected with HIV	Adults (15–49) prevalence (%)	Adult (15+) and child deaths due to AIDS
Sub-Saharan Africa				
2005	24.5 million	2.7 million	6.1	2.0 million
2003	23.5 million	2.6 million	6.2	1.9 million
North Africa and Middle East				
2005	440 000	64 000	0.2	37 000
2003	380 000	54 000	0.2	34 000
Asia				
2005	8.3 million	930 000	0.4	600 000
2003	7.6 million	860 000	0.4	500 000
Oceania				
2005	78 000	7 200	0.3	3 400
2003	66 000	9 000	0.3	2 300
Latin America				
2005	1.6 million	140 000	0.5	59 000

Table 1. (*Continued*)

Country	Adults (15+) and children living with HIV	Adults (15+) and children newly infected with HIV	Adults (15–49) prevalence (%)	Adult (15+) and child deaths due to AIDS
2003	1.4 million	130 000	0.5	51 000
Caribbean				
2005	330 000	37 000	1.6	27 000
2003	310 000	34 000	1.5	28 000
Eastern Europe and Central Asia				
2005	1.5 million	220 000	0.8	53 000
2003	1.1 million	160 000	0.6	28 000
North America, Western and Central Europe				
2005	2.0 million	65 000	0.5	30 000
2003	1.8 million	65 000	0.5	30 000
TOTAL				
2005	38.6 million	4.1 million	1.0	2.8 million
2003	36.2 million	3.9 million	1.0	2.6 million

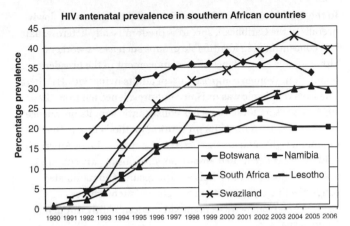

HIV antenatal prevalence in southern African countries

Legend:
◆ Botswana ■ Namibia
▲ South Africa ━ Lesotho
✕ Swaziland

Y-axis: Percentatge prevalence (0 to 45)
X-axis: 1990 1991 1992 1993 1994 1995 1996 1997 1998 1999 2000 2001 2002 2003 2004 2005 2006

2. **Southern African epidemics: HIV prevalence in antenatal clinic patients**

1.1% in 2002 and falling back to 0.9% in 2005, although increases in prevalence are being reported from some specific groups such as migrant men.

In East Africa, prevalence peaked and is declining. Behavioural data show this is due to increased condom use in casual relationships; reduction in numbers of partners; and delayed sexual debut. The greatest reduction is in Uganda, which, in the 1980s, was the global epicentre of the epidemic: at the peak in 1990, HIV prevalence may have been 31% among pregnant women; it was believed to be just 4.7% in this group in 2002.

In North Africa and the Middle East, although there is little evidence of HIV, there is concern about high risk factors. Sexual intercourse is the dominant form of transmission but there are signs of spread among drug users. Stigma and discrimination are particularly marked here and mean the epidemic remains hidden.

In the Caribbean and Latin America, numbers are rising slowly overall. In the Caribbean, spread is predominantly heterosexual and concentrated in identifiable groups such as sex workers, although there is evidence of slow movement to the broader population. Women comprise 51% of adults living with HIV here. The worst epidemic was in Haiti, but prevalence fell from 6.2% in 1993 to 3.8% in 2006. Cuba has consistently kept its prevalence very low, less than 0.1%. Its prevention methods flew in the face of human rights and are discussed in Chapter 7. Latin America's epidemic is concentrated among populations at particular risk, and the majority of infections are the result of contaminated drug-injecting equipment or sex between men, whereas in Central America, the virus is spread predominantly through heterosexual sex.

In Eastern Europe, the number of HIV infections, being driven primarily by IDUs, has risen dramatically, reaching 1.5 million at the end of 2005. Prior to 1990, there were few infections, and most of those affected were foreigners. The most serious epidemic proportionately is in Ukraine. Here, between 1987 and 1994, some 39 million tests were done and only 398 cases of HIV were detected, of which 54% were foreign. The epidemic took off in 1995, when 1,489 infections were identified, of which 99.4% were Ukrainian and 68.6% were IDUs. By the end of 2005, an estimated 410,000 people were infected, an adult prevalence rate of 1.4%. Ukraine's epidemic continues to expand, and newly registered HIV infections increased by 25% in 2002. The Russian Federation has the highest number of infections: an estimated 940,000 people. Between 1.5 and 3 million Russians are believed to inject drugs (1% to 2% of the entire population). In the Baltic states of Belarus and Moldova, transmission is increasing, although overall the numbers remain low. Intravenous drug use accounts for the largest proportion of newly reported infections but sexual transmission is slowly gaining ground.

HIV prevalence is low (less than 0.3%) in most of Central Asia and the Caucasus, though numbers are rising. The epidemic is recent: in Uzbekistan, reported infections rose from 28 in 1999 to 2,016 in 2004. Given that the epidemic is located in core transmitter groups – IDUs and sex workers – it might be halted with prevention strategies concentrating on those most at risk. However, coverage is low: 10% of sex workers, fewer than 8% of IDUs, and 4% of men who have sex with men are reached by prevention messages.

In Asia, HIV infection levels are low, but large populations translate this to huge numbers of HIV-positive people. Some 8.3 million people are infected here, the largest number in India. The pace and severity of Asia's epidemics vary. Some countries responded quickly and effectively, while others are experiencing expanding epidemics and need to mount responses. Indonesia, Nepal, Vietnam, and several provinces in China, Bangladesh, Laos, Pakistan, and the Philippines have extremely low levels of HIV. HIV spread in China is attributable to IDUs, paid sex, and pooling of blood among donors for transfusion. In India, Indonesia, Myanmar, and Vietnam, drug use is an important driver.

Thailand seemed set to experience a large epidemic, between late 1987 and mid-1988 prevalence rose from 0 to more than 30% among IDUs in Bangkok. Prevalence among sex workers was between 1% and 5% in various locations in 1989, but in the city of Chiang Mai it was 44%. The government reaction was immediate and forceful: efforts were mounted to promote condom use, reduce risky behaviour, treat STIs, and provide care. A cornerstone of the response was the '100% condom programme', which required consistent condom use in brothels. Early indicators of success were increased condom use from 14% to over 90% by 1992 in brothels, and a decrease in episodes of male STIs at government clinics from 200,000 in 1989 to 20,000 in

1995. HIV prevalence among pregnant women peaked at 2.35% in 1995, and declined to 1.18% in 2003. Prevalence among military conscripts decreased from 4% in 1993 to 0.5% in 2003. However, the HIV prevalence among IDUs remained high at 33% in 2003.

The epidemic is largely under control in the developed world. In 2005, there were 65,000 new infections in this region, raising the number of people with HIV to 2 million. Widespread access to life-prolonging ART meant that the number of AIDS deaths was just 30,000 in 2005. Sex between men and, to a lesser extent, intravenous drug use are the predominant routes of transmission, but patterns are changing and new populations are being affected through unprotected heterosexual intercourse. In the United States, the epidemic is increasingly located among African Americans (over 50% of new HIV diagnoses in recent years have been made in this group) and is affecting greater numbers of women (African American women account for 72% of new HIV diagnoses). In Canada, indigenous populations are disproportionately infected. In 12 Western European countries with data for new infections, HIV diagnoses in people infected through heterosexual contact increased by 122% between 1997 and 2002, and most originated from countries with generalized epidemics in sub-Saharan Africa or the Caribbean.

Key features of the epidemic

A number of points can be drawn from this brief survey. There are differences between and within countries in terms of the size, timing, and location of the epidemics, they are not homogeneous; prevalence rates have risen to levels believed impossible a decade ago; and the epidemic does not respect national borders.

The timing varies. Where the epidemic was reported early, such as in Uganda and Thailand, by 1990 HIV prevalence had peaked and was declining; whereas in Southern Africa, HIV did not begin spreading among the general population until the 1990s, and in the former Soviet Union, a rapid increase in prevalence began in the late 1990s. In some countries HIV has plateaued, although deaths may have been simply replaced by new infections. In other settings the small numbers of infections in particularly vulnerable populations are remaining stable. Given the 'right' change in circumstances, a broader spread might occur.

The maximum possible extent of the epidemic is uncertain. In 2002, UNAIDS, reporting on Southern Africa, noted that HIV prevalence had reached levels 'considerably higher than had previously been thought possible'. There is a 'natural limit' beyond which prevalence will not grow, when everyone who is likely to be infected has been. The highest national prevalence recorded so far was Swaziland's 42.6% among antenatal clinic patients in 2004; in 2006, prevalence had fallen to 39.2%.

Location refers both to physical geographic (spatial) location and particular population groups. There are epidemic hotspots. For example, in Brazil national prevalence is well below 1%, but in some cities infection levels of over 60% have been reported among IDUs. African prevalence is higher in urban areas, near major transport routes, and at trading centres than in the rural areas, and some of the highest localized prevalence rates have been recorded at border posts.

Sometimes clearly defined groups can be identified, usually those on the margins of society and who face legal or social stigmatization: sex workers, drug users, and men who have sex with men. In China's central provinces many cases are due to the sale of blood. Peasants sold their blood, the plasma was extracted, and what was left was pooled and transfused back, a practice that prevented anaemia in the donors but ensured rapid spread of HIV, hepatitis, malaria, and other blood-borne diseases. In other provinces of China there is primarily an IDU-driven epidemic.

The international dimension of the epidemic is not always appreciated. It can be illustrated with two examples. In South East Asia, the 'golden triangle' is the main opium-producing area and covers the mountainous region where Myanmar, Laos, and Thailand meet and has links into southern China, the states of eastern India, and northern Vietnam. Drugs are a major illegal export and the area is home to many addicts and hence infected people. If the golden triangle were a country, it would have a high prevalence and be a major source of concern to 'its' government.

The second example concerns the UK, where, since 1996, there have been 29,357 HIV diagnoses. Year after year the number of new diagnoses has risen steadily, from 2,014 in 2000, to 4,474 for 2003, the last year for which there are complete data (the Health Protection Agency reports 4,287 cases in 2004 but expects numbers to rise as more data are received). The vast majority of new HIV infections worldwide – 92.5% – were heterosexually contracted. Of these, 78.6% were infected in the developing world, most in Southern and Eastern Africa. Some of these people are political or economic refugees, others have been recruited to work in fields with skills shortages.

Migration and refugee flows are contributing to the continued increases in HIV prevalence in many European countries. It is a complex and difficult problem, and reaffirms HIV/AIDS as a global dilemma even for countries where prevalence is low.

Key concepts: prevalence and incidence

Prevalence and incidence are key concepts in epidemiology and are important for understanding the spread of HIV and associated data. Prevalence is the absolute number of people infected. The prevalence rate is the proportion of the population that has a disease at a particular time (or averaged over a period of time). With HIV, prevalence rates are given as a percentage of a specific segment of the population, for example adults aged between 15 and 65, antenatal clinic patients, blood donors, or an 'at risk' group. HIV prevalence data come from surveys: in the early years, surveys were done among blood donors, STI clinic patients, people with TB, and pregnant women.

Incidence is the number of new infections over a given period of time. The incidence rate is the number per specified unit of population (this can be per 1,000, per 10,000, or per million for rare diseases) and period of time (in the case of cholera, for example, this can be per day or week). Measuring HIV incidence is complex and expensive.

People infected with HIV remain so for the rest of their lives; the only way they leave the pool of HIV infections is to die. This means the prevalence can continue rising even after the incidence has peaked, and the introduction of ART makes understanding data more complex as people live longer. This is explored in Table 2. In this example, incidence peaks in year 6, and prevalence continues to rise, then the introduction of ART in year 9 means that it rises even more rapidly.

Where information comes from

In the early days AIDS cases caught the headlines and provided an indicator of the spread. The number of people falling ill and dying rose relentlessly; no one knew who was at risk or how far the disease would spread. Each country counted the number of AIDS cases and sent this information to the World Health Organization (WHO), which then reported on the state of the global pandemic.

AIDS case data are no longer routinely collected, except in well-resourced countries. The most commonly used and reported information is HIV prevalence; the estimated number

Table 2. Incidence and prevalence

Year	Population	Incidence (actual)	Incidence rate per 1000	Prevalence	Prevalence rate (%)	Deaths of infected people	Comments
1	9 750	0		0			Year zero
2	10 000	50	5	50	0.5		
3	10 250	50	4.8	100	0.97		Slow increase
4	10 500	150	14.3	250	2.3		Exponential
5	10 750	550	51	750	6.9	200	
6	11 000	700	68	1150	10.5	300	Peak incidence
7	11 250	650	57.7	1400	12.4	400	
8	11 400	600	52.6	1550	13.6	450	
9	11 400	400	35	1750	15.4	200	ART introduced
10	11 300	300	26.5	1850	16.4	200	

Data sources

The best source of information, other than looking at each country individually, is UNAIDS, which produces a biannual report including a statistical annex. These data are mainly based on what is collected and reported by each country. This gives rise to problems, and in some instances, we simply do not know what the situation is. There are few data from states in conflict, such as the Democratic Republic of the Congo or Sudan, or those without a functioning government to collect, collate, and disseminate information, for example Afghanistan and Somalia. Data may simply not be credible due to inefficiency and government failure. An example is Nigeria: data reported by UNAIDS in 2006 for Nigeria came from surveys done in 2001, at only 10 urban and 70 rural sites. In Zimbabwe it is hard to believe reliable HIV data are being collected as the health system is overstretched and the economy is collapsing.

Data are sensitive. UNAIDS was unable to publish an estimate of the numbers of people infected with HIV in India in 2004 as the government would not agree to a figure (although they were allowed to put in an estimate: 2,200,000 to 7,600,000 infections). In July 2007, new estimates were released by the Indian Government, UNAIDS, and the WHO, putting the figure at between 2 and 3.1 million infections. For political reasons, the UN finds it difficult to make negative comments on the quality of the data with which they are presented.

The 2006 UNAIDS report notes the global estimates of people living with HIV/AIDS are lower than previously reported. This is because of genuine declines in prevalence in some settings and because new data are available from population-based surveys.

The 2006 report looks at all adults, whereas previously only those aged 15 to 49 were included. More HIV-infected people are living beyond 50, and ART will increase this further.

of infections; and the number of orphans due to AIDS. HIV prevalence is given as the percentage of those infected of all adults (until recently this was given as people between the ages of 15 and 49).

The most consistent prevalence data come from women in antenatal clinic (ANC) surveys. Originally this population was chosen because they provided the best sample: blood was routinely taken for other tests; the women had been sexually active; and the surveys could be done on an anonymous basis, meaning the sample could not be linked to individual women, so informed consent was not required.

ANC data give a reasonable picture of the epidemic provided biases are recognized. The main biases are that men are excluded; younger women are over-represented (as they are more sexually active and likely to fall pregnant); HIV-positive and older women are under-represented as HIV infection and age reduce fertility; and surveys usually draw on women attending public antenatal clinics. This last point means women who are too poor to access the government clinics and also those who get private health care will be excluded.

Once data are available, it is possible to estimate the number and percentage of all women, men, and adults who are infected, as well as the number of children who will be born HIV positive, by using models that adjust for the biases. Some models are in the public domain and accessible through the Internet.

New data are becoming available through population-based surveys of HIV prevalence, which collect nationally representative information on HIV prevalence and provide data on characteristics associated with infection and risk. Most have been done as part of the Demographic and Health Surveys (DHS). Since 2001 there have been 13 surveys carried out and published by the US-based Macro International Inc., and a further 20 are in various stages of completion at the time of writing in 2007. A comparison between the recent DHS results and UNAIDS estimates showed that in three cases UNAIDS estimated adult prevalence was higher, in four instances lower, and in the remaining six the rates were the same. Both DHS and ANC data sets can be used provided they are treated with care.

Two population surveys in South Africa were carried out for the Nelson Mandela Foundation by the Human Sciences Research Council, in 2002 and 2005. The entire population, except children under 2, were sampled. The 2002 survey found a prevalence rate of 17.7% among women aged 15–49. By 2005, it had increased to 20.2%. The survey allows us to locate the epidemic by age and gender, as shown in Figure 3. This figure is typical of the

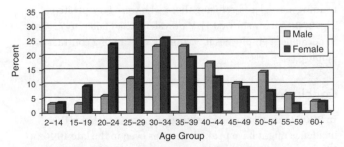

3. **HIV prevalence by sex and age group, South Africa, 2005**

heterosexual epidemics. If a graph of prevalence were drawn for Russia, it would show more men than women infected, as their epidemic is being driven by IDUs.

In addition to surveys among ANC patients, specific risk groups, and population-based studies, there are other data sources. Most common are of specific occupations such as the military, teachers, health workers, and employees of particular companies (although these may not be in the public domain). A survey of teachers in South Africa in 2005 showed HIV prevalence was highest in the 25–34 age group (21.4%), followed by the 35–44 age group (12.8%). This has policy implications, as teachers are crucial for economic and social development. In Nigeria, HIV prevalence among army troops was estimated to be less than 1% in 1989/90, it increased to 5% in 1997, and 10% in 1999. Among Nigerian troops in Sierra Leone, prevalence increased from 7% after one year to more than 15% after three years of duty in the operational area.

In Botswana, Debswana, the diamond-mining company, carried out its first survey in 1999 and found HIV prevalence across all employees was 28.8%. The company decided to provide ART for staff and spouses, re-target their prevention programmes, and require 'AIDS compliance' from contractors. They maintained their policy of testing scholarship applicants for long-term training abroad and refusing those who were HIV positive. The 2003 survey showed HIV prevalence had fallen to 22.6%: in permanent employees it was 19.9% and among contract employees 28.3%.

Conclusion

In 2006 there were cautious suggestions that global HIV incidence might have peaked, perhaps even in the late 1990s. The 2006 UNAIDS epidemic report revised the global number of people living with HIV slightly downwards from its 2005 figures. However, HIV data must be seen against a backdrop of the three curves (see Figure 1). In 2002, it was estimated that HIV/AIDS caused 4.9% of deaths globally and a quarter of all deaths from infectious and parasitic diseases. The WHO estimates that in 2015 AIDS will still cause one in six deaths in Africa.

Chapter 2
How HIV/AIDS works and scientific responses

AIDS appeared at a time when the world was growing ever more interconnected, one of the reasons it spread so rapidly. It also came at a point of unprecedented scientific advance and confidence. The eradication of smallpox in 1977, advances in virology and immunology and in a range of other medical disciplines had given rise to optimism about what science and medicine could do.

Although there was the science available to understand its origins and the mechanisms of HIV and AIDS, it soon became clear there was to be no medical or scientific silver bullet. Preventing HIV transmission and successfully treating patients needs more than scientific solutions. The epidemic has found its most fertile locations in parts of the world where there is poverty and inequity, especially where this is gendered. Dealing with this disease means understanding the science and then looking beyond it.

How the virus works

There are two main sub-types of the virus: HIV-1 and HIV-2, the latter being harder to transmit and slower-acting. Both originate in simian (monkey) immunodeficiency viruses (SIV) found in Africa. The source of HIV-1 was chimpanzees in Central Africa, while HIV-2 derived in West Africa from sooty mangabey monkeys. How and when the virus crossed the species barrier continue to be sources of speculation and historical interest. Current thinking is that the epidemic had its origins through chimpanzee and monkey blood entering people's bodies possibly during the butchering of bush meat in the 1930s.

Viruses have been described as 'a piece of nucleic acid surrounded by bad news'. A virus is genetic material covered with a coat of protein molecules. Viruses do not have cell walls, are parasitic, and can only replicate by entering host cells. They have few genes compared with other organisms: HIV has fewer than 10 genes; the smallpox virus has between 200 and 400 genes; the smallest bacterium has 5,000 to 10,000 genes; and humans have about 30,000 genes.

The genetic material of life forms, including most viruses, is deoxyribonucleic acid (DNA). This contains the genetic instructions specifying the biological development of cellular life. Some viruses, including HIV, have ribonucleic acid (RNA) as their genetic material, and are called retroviruses (scientifically, *retroviridae*). HIV also belongs in the family of viruses known as lentiviruses, which means slow-acting. In humans, lentiviruses result in diseases that develop over a long period, many affecting the immune system and brain.

HIV has to invade cells to reproduce. Within these cells, it produces more virus particles by converting viral RNA into DNA in the cell and then making many RNA copies. The conversion is done through an enzyme called reverse transcriptase. The switch from RNA to DNA and back to RNA is significant and makes combating HIV difficult. Each time it occurs there is a possibility of errors and the virus mutating. This is made more likely because reverse transcriptase lacks the normal 'proofreading' that occurs with DNA replication. Once formed, the copies or virus particles break out of the cell, destroying it and infecting other cells.

The mutation of the virus means various sub-types or clades of virus have evolved. Identifying clades allows scientists and epidemiologists to track the spread of infection across the world. Type B is the main clade in the USA, type C in Southern Africa, while in East Africa, A and D are most common. The greatest variety is in West Central Africa.

Mutation means the virus can outwit human responses, both our biological response and the technology we deploy through drug development. Individual human immune systems fight infections, and we can pass this resistance and response on to the next generations. However, HIV attacks the cells of the immune system and, in particular, CD4 cells. There are two main types of CD4 cells. The prime target is CD4 T cells which organize the body's overall immune response to foreign bodies and infections. The virus also attacks immune cells called macrophages which engulf foreign invaders in the body and ensure the immune system will recognize them in the future. Once the virus has penetrated the wall of the CD4 cell it is safe because it has become part of the immune system. The biological response of 'herd immunity', where the ability to fight an infection is passed on, or succeeding generations are 'selected' because they are resistant to a disease, does not yet occur with HIV.

Virus particles lie dormant in the cells until their replication is triggered. The trigger is not fully understood but could be an infection such as TB, or the deterioration of the immune system. The process of viral insertion, transcription, and particle expulsion is shown in Figure 4.

Our technological response is limited. The virus mutates and becomes resistant to drugs. For an individual, this means the drug combination they take should be tailored to the variant of virus with which they are infected. A person developing drug-resistant HIV infection in the rich world requires costly tests, sophisticated

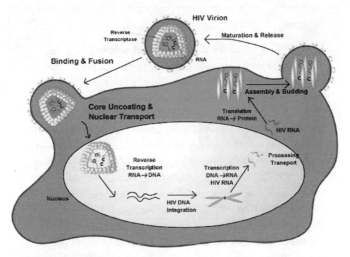

4. The HIV life cycle

laboratory facilities, and drug combinations; in the poor world, it is usually a death sentence. At the population level, drug-resistant infections have long-term ramifications; if they spread, treatment becomes much more difficult and expensive for everyone.

HIV mutation may mean it becomes less of a killer, but equally it could become more robust and easily transmitted. Virologists monitor the virus and its changes to ensure we are warned of new developments. While it is generally understood that HIV infection is for life, what is often not appreciated is that an HIV-infected person can be re-infected with new strains of the virus, damaging their prospects for survival. Effectively, such individuals get 'super-infections'.

When a person is newly infected, they sero-convert – this means the virus has taken hold in the body and it (or its antibodies) will be detectable by an HIV test. During this period, an infected

25

Testing

Most HIV tests look for the presence of antibodies to the virus rather than detecting the virus itself: if a person has antibodies, they have the virus. The most common test for antibodies is the enzyme-linked immunosorbent assay (ELISA), which is cheap and simple to perform. Initially, HIV could only be detected using blood samples. The South African and the DHS surveys described in Chapter 1 collected people's blood on absorbent paper by pricking a finger, heel, or ear. This is invasive, as people don't like having blood taken, but it is as simple as the process many diabetics go through daily to assess their blood-sugar levels. However, there are now tests that can identify the antibodies in saliva and other body fluids and they are quick and easy to use, especially in the context of population surveys. Tests have also been developed to estimate how recently a person has been infected, giving a measure of incidence.

Although the indirect tests such as ELISA are cheaper and quicker than testing for the virus itself, testing for the virus is sometimes preferable and involves a process called polymerase chain reaction (PCR). This uses a technique by which DNA from a cell can be replicated to a point when it can be measured. Both ELISAs and PCRs are also used for detection of diseases other than HIV.

person may experience a flu-like illness and will have very high viral loads, that is the number of virus particles in the blood or body fluids, especially semen or vaginal secretions, will be high.

However, there is a 'window' period when a person may be infected and infectious but the virus is not yet detectable, meaning HIV tests are not completely reliable for new infections, and blood supply safety cannot be guaranteed. In the period immediately after infection, a person will be very infectious. This is of epidemiological importance. The more people there are in the early stage of infection, the greater the chance of exposure and infection, thus the epidemic builds up its own momentum. Infectivity also rises as the disease progresses and the viral load increases.

The window period is followed by the long incubation stage. During this phase, the viruses and the cells they attack are reproducing rapidly and are being wiped out as quickly by each other. Every day up to 5% of the body's CD4 cells (about 2,000 million cells) may be destroyed by approximately 10 billion new virus particles. Eventually, the virus destroys immune cells more quickly than they can be replaced. A healthy CD4 cell count is normally over 1,000 cells per mm³ of blood. As infection progresses, this number falls, as shown in Figure 5.

The World Health Organization recognizes four stages in HIV disease progression. Stage 1 is asymptomatic infection, when the CD4 count is normally greater than 500 per mm³ of blood.

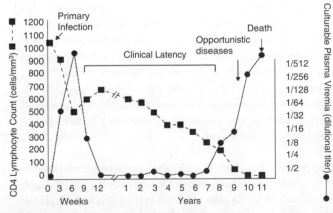

5. Viral load and CD4 cell counts over time

Stage 2 is when the count is between 350 and 499 per mm^3, and symptoms might include some mild weight loss, fungal infections, and herpes zoster (shingles). When the CD4 cell count falls below 350, in stage 3, a person has advanced immunosuppression with opportunistic infections, fevers, severe weight loss, diarrhoea, candidiasis (infection with a yeast-like fungus that causes thrush), and possibly TB. Stage 4, AIDS, occurs when there are fewer than 200 CD4 cells per mm^3 of blood and the person is seriously ill with diseases such as TB which may spread beyond the lungs, *Pneumocystis carinii* and other pneumonias, the parasitic disease toxoplasmosis, and meningitis.

A few people may experience symptoms of disease with CD4 counts above 200, while others show no symptoms with CD4 counts below 200. Generally though, infections will increase in frequency, severity, and duration until the person dies. The CD4 count is one of the measures used by physicians in deciding when to begin drug therapy.

Transmission

HIV is found in all body fluids of an infected person, although in minimal quantities in sweat, tears, and saliva. Exposure to blood or blood products carries the maximum risk of infection. This is why there is so much concern around blood safety and hygiene in health care settings, and why there are high levels of transmission among drug users who share syringes. However, sexual intercourse is the most common source of transmission: 75–85% of people are infected this way. This includes both homosexual and heterosexual intercourse, though globally heterosexual intercourse predominates.

The virus can be passed from infected mothers to their infants by crossing the placenta, during the birth process, and through breast milk. Reducing the risk prior to or during birth is simple: in most resource-poor settings, the drug nevirapine is used, which lowers mother-to-child transmission from about 25% to between 8% and 17%. The drug is cheap and easily administered, with one dose for the mother prior to delivery and a dose for the infant after birth. Where affordable, more complex treatments, including ART, are offered, and are so successful that few babies are born with HIV infection. If mothers have access to clean water and infant feeding formula, then bottle-feeding means HIV will not be transmitted through breast milk. However, in many settings this is not the case, and work at the University of KwaZulu-Natal has shown that where formula and clean water are not available, babies of women who exclusively breast-feed are substantially less likely to be infected than infants who are given both formula and breast milk.

The comparative efficiency of different modes of transmission is shown in Table 3. The chance of infection varies with stage of disease, and the viral load is crucial. Also important is the state of the immune system, health, and nutritional status of the exposed person. One benefit of ART is that it reduces the viral load, making a person on treatment much less infectious. There is a debate as to whether treatment will increase or reduce the scale of the epidemic. Reduced viral loads reduce infectivity, but the infected person is around for longer, and may be more sexually active; on the other hand, people on treatment may want to protect themselves and others. There is no clear evidence on this yet.

Treatment

The period from infection to illness is, on average, about eight years. This can be extended with basic lifestyle changes; a person who eats properly, does not smoke, take drugs, or excessive amounts of alcohol, and gets regular exercise will live a longer and healthier life. Immune system boosters, including some indigenous and herbal preparations, can help prevent opportunistic infections and prolong life.

Table 3. Routes of exposure and risk of infection

Infection route	Risk of infection
Sexual transmission	
Female-to-male transmission	1:700 to 1:3000
Male-to-female transmission	1:200 to 1:2000
Male-to-male transmission	1:10 to 1:1600
Fellatio	0 to 6:100
Parenteral transmission	
Transfusion of infected blood	95:100
Needle-sharing	1:150
Needle stick	1:200
Needle stick/AZT PEP	1:10000
Transmission from mother to infant	
Without AZT treatment	1:4
With AZT treatment	Less than 1:10

There has been considerable debate on the importance of nutrition. A WHO-led consultation in Durban in 2005 confirmed that infected people have greater calorific needs. Asymptomatic adults and children require 10% more energy from their diet than uninfected adults or children, and adults who have become ill need 20 to 30% more energy, while sick children require 50 to 100% more. There is, as yet, no evidence of greater protein requirements among infected people, and the relationships between micronutrient supplementation and HIV/AIDS need more investigation. Complicating factors are that people suffering from HIV/AIDS often experience loss of appetite, inability to eat due to infections of the mouth and throat, and failure to properly digest food. Additionally, the loss of labour and income that results from family members becoming ill may lead to there being less food available in the household (see Chapter 5).

As the CD4 cell count falls and the immune system is compromised, the infected person experiences 'opportunistic' infections – that is, infections that would rarely affect or cause serious symptoms in people whose immune systems were healthy. Most can be treated, and the role of prophylaxis is important. An antibiotic such as cotrimoxazole prevents *Pneumocystis carinii* infections and other bacterial pneumonias, toxoplasmosis, and salmonella bacteraemia, and tuberculosis can be prevented with isoniazid. These treatments are cheap and effective, but do not address the underlying HIV infection.

Eventually ART is needed. These drugs reduce viral activity, allow the immune system to recover, and prolong and improve quality of life. As an illustration of their effectiveness, in the USA by 1991, HIV was the leading cause of death among adults aged 25 to 44, and rates reached close to 40 deaths per 100,000 by 1995. The introduction of ART in 1996 meant mortality plummeted, so that by 2000, it had fallen to about 10 per 100,000. Patients who had resigned themselves to death, cashed in life insurance policies, and given up employment found themselves granted a new lease of life – so dramatic it became known as the 'Lazarus syndrome'.

The first effective drug was azidothymidine, known as AZT with the trade name Retrovir. This had short-term benefits but resistance to the drug in the body developed rapidly. It was found that combinations of drugs, acting in different places and on different stages of the viral replication cycle (shown in Figure 4) were most effective, and the standard treatment is currently triple therapy using three different drugs. In the wealthy world, the combination of drugs will be tailored to the needs of the patient and even the variant of the virus with which they are infected. These do not eliminate the virus from a patient's body, and reservoirs of infection remain. If treatment ceases, the virus will emerge and begin replication again, therefore current therapies have to be taken for life.

In resource-poor settings the combination of drugs offered usually includes, as a first line of treatment, two from a class called non-nucleoside reverse transcriptase inhibitors (NNRTIs) and one nucleoside reverse transcriptase inhibitor (NRTI). There is evidence suggesting this first-line therapy provides about five years of healthy life before resistance develops. When this occurs, a second line of treatment must be adopted to prolong life. The WHO recommends that second-line therapy include two NRTIs and a third class of drug called protease inhibitors (PIs).

All the drugs used to treat HIV/AIDS are complex and expensive (particularly PIs, which also require special handling – refrigeration). They are also toxic. Not all patients can tolerate them, and not all drugs will work for an individual patient. The more the combinations and dosages can be adapted to the individual, the better their prognosis. Additionally, few drugs are available in paediatric formulations, which means that infected infants and children have to take adaptations of adult drugs (although this is changing).

There is a debate as to the best time to begin the ART regimen. Early treatment prevents damage to the body caused by high and prolonged viral loads, but decreases options if resistance builds up. The WHO guidelines, somewhat unhelpfully, say:

'the optimum time to commence ART is before patients become unwell or present with their first opportunistic infection'. This assumes that people know their HIV status, and most don't. The guidelines state treatment should be considered when the CD4 cell count falls below 350 and certainly started before it is 200 or lower. Where there are laboratory services available, the viral load (the number of virus particles in a person's blood) can be monitored and, if it rises above 55,000 copies per millilitre, treatment should start.

Where resources are limited, the tendency is to treat more conservatively. In South Africa, for example, national guidelines are that a person with a CD4 cell count of less than 200 should be put on ART. In most African and Asian countries this is the standard of care in public health settings.

Cost is a factor. In affluent countries, where physicians tailor combinations of drugs, the total cost of treatment per patient is between US$ 850 and US$ 1,500 per month (this includes drugs, laboratory tests, and health care staff). In 2007, the cheapest combination of drugs in the developing world was US$ 94 per patient per year. This, with associated costs of laboratory testing and health care worker time, means the lowest possible price for first-line treatment would be about US$ 250 annually.

Western pharmaceutical companies are the main source of new drugs, but cheaper generic versions come from developing world manufacturers, mainly in India and Thailand, with South Africa and Brazil being recent entrants into drug manufacturing. The major purchasers of drugs are international development agencies, the American Presidential Emergency Plan for AIDS Relief (PEPFAR), the Global Fund for HIV/AIDS, TB and Malaria (Global Fund), and national treatment programmes. The prices paid vary greatly from country to country, and even within a country depending on who does the purchasing.

Despite recent price reductions, affordability and access remain an issue for most people in poor countries. In Uganda combined public and private spending on all health care is estimated at only US$ 38 per capita per year. The cost of ART drugs alone is US$ 28 per month, and this excludes clinical consultations, monitoring, tests, and drugs for opportunistic infections. Only wealthy people can afford medicines, and even they have to make difficult decisions about whether and when to spend their household resources on drugs. In poor parts of the world, most people are treated in public health facilities and treatment is funded by international donors.

It is not only the cost of drugs that creates problems of access: poor people may not be able to afford transport to clinics, and since some drugs must be taken with food, the effectiveness of treatment may be diminished if patients are malnourished. Poverty therefore affects adherence to and success of treatment.

Tuberculosis and HIV

The issue of TB and HIV is not fully understood outside the medical arena. While most diseases that affect HIV-positive people are not a threat to others, TB is an exception. The WHO says that HIV/AIDS and TB are so closely connected the terms 'co-epidemic' or 'dual epidemic' can be used to describe the relationship, and HIV and TB have variously been referred to as 'the terrible twins' and 'Bonnie and Clyde'. Each disease speeds up progress of the other: TB shortens the survival time of people with HIV/AIDS, killing up to half of all AIDS patients worldwide; HIV-positive people have increased likelihood of acquiring new TB infection, are more likely to develop active TB, and relapse if previously treated. Having HIV makes the diagnosis of TB more complex, and prophylactic and curative treatment for TB in HIV-positive people is more costly and problematic.

34

The WHO recommends that TB patients be offered voluntary counselling and testing for HIV, while people who are HIV infected should be tested for TB and treated or given prophylaxis. Ideally, TB patients should have their disease brought under control before being put on ART.

TB infections are spreading at the rate of one person per second. Every year 8–10 million people catch the disease and 2 million die from it. About 2 billion people carry the bacteria that cause TB, but most never develop the active disease; around 10% of infected people actually develop symptoms, although this proportion is rising as the number of people with weakened immune systems grows. Most cases of TB can be treated, and the DOTs regime (Directly Observed Treatment, short course) has dramatically raised cure rates. However, as with HIV, the number of drug-resistant cases is growing, and up to 50 million people worldwide may be infected with drug-resistant TB. Treating multi-drug-resistant (MDR) TB takes up to two years (as opposed to six months for DOTs) and is more complex and expensive.

Towards the end of 2006, there were reports from South Africa of an outbreak of extensively drug-resistant (XDR) TB, a form that is extremely difficult to treat as few drugs are effective. In one hospital in Tugela Ferry, of 542 TB patients, 53 had XDR TB, and 52 of these patients died within weeks of being tested. Of the 53 patients, 44 were tested for HIV and all were positive. While this outbreak caught the attention of the media, in March of 2006 the CDC and WHO had already reported XDR TB from 17 countries.

The links between TB and HIV have the potential to make HIV a broader public health issue. Exposure to TB is more difficult to control since the bacteria that cause it are airborne. In settings where large numbers of people are HIV positive, a serious TB epidemic may occur with consequent increased illness and death for those infected, as well as increased risks to the broader general population. This has been largely ignored or skated over by public health professions and the media. There is a growing recognition that TB and HIV programmes need to work together to achieve effective control of the diseases. Furthermore, the outbreak of XDR TB reveals the weaknesses in existing public health and disease control programmes.

Biomedical interventions: vaccines, microbicides, and circumcision

The ultimate scientific solution to HIV would be a cheap, effective vaccine. Since Edward Jenner vaccinated an eight-year-old boy against smallpox in 1796, vaccines have been seen as a way of eliminating diseases in populations. The first disease to be eradicated worldwide was indeed smallpox – the last 'wild' case occurring in 1977. Vaccines now provide protection against a range of childhood diseases including measles, mumps, and rubella.

Unfortunately progress towards a vaccine for HIV is slow. The International AIDS Vaccine Initiative (IAVI) notes that there are difficult scientific questions impeding development of a vaccine. There are also economic issues: vaccine development is resource-intensive and, although most research is conducted in the rich world, there is little commercial incentive – the market is limited and risks are high. When a vaccine is developed, there will be questions about its efficacy. What level of protection would it offer, and for what duration? Would one inoculation be sufficient, or would boosters be required? There is a danger that a vaccine might give people a false sense of security and increase the spread of HIV because of continued or even increased unsafe sexual activity.

A microbicide is a substance (gel or foam) that could be inserted into the vagina prior to intercourse, to kill viruses and bacteria. This would provide women with protection they could control.

Development of microbicides has been incomprehensibly slow. Unlike vaccines, the reason is not primarily scientific but to do with the markets and gender inequity – the main market would be poor women in poor countries who have little spending power. Nonetheless, there are currently 60 substances being studied as potential microbicides and five tested for safety, and it is possible that, should safety and efficacy be established, a microbicide could be available by 2012.

Research into vaccines and microbicides is increasingly supported by a number of philanthropists, including the Bill and Melinda Gates Foundation. While this support is welcomed and important, there is a danger of seeing money and science as providing the solutions to the epidemic. Both interventions are some years away, and even when they do become available they will be only part of the solution.

Early analysis by Australian demographers Jack and Pat Caldwell suggested there were links between male circumcision and patterns of HIV. The science is clear. In uncircumcised men, the area under the foreskin and the foreskin itself contain many of the cells the virus binds to (the Langerhans' cells), and the skin or mucosal surface of the foreskin is more easily penetrated. Circumcised men are less likely to contract and pass on other sexually transmitted infections.

In South Africa, a study at Orange Farm outside Johannesburg suggested circumcision could be 60% protective against HIV infection. The study was stopped in November 2004 after interim analysis showed 'the protection effect' of male circumcision was so high that it would have been unethical to continue. Similarly, in December 2006, the US National Institute of Allergy and Infectious Diseases (NIAID) halted two trials of adult male circumcision because data showed medically performed circumcision greatly reduced male risk of HIV infection. In Kisumu, Kenya, there was a 53% reduction of HIV acquisition in circumcised men, and in Rakai, Uganda, HIV acquisition was reduced by 48%.

In March 2007, WHO and UNAIDS issued their conclusions and recommendations on male circumcision for HIV prevention. They found that male circumcision, without doubt, reduces female-to-male HIV transmission and should be recognized as an important additional prevention strategy. While access to circumcision should be made available for men and adolescent boys, it is less complicated and risky for infants, and so neonatal circumcision should be promoted.

However, circumcision raises similar questions to vaccination – would those who are circumcised behave in a more risky manner because they believe themselves to be protected? There are also gender issues. It is only male circumcision that is protective; there is no evidence to suggest that male circumcision reduces transmission from infected men to uninfected women. Clearly, though, if fewer men are infected then their female partners are also less likely to be infected. At present, the major determinant of circumcision is religion; it could, in the era of AIDS, become a medical rather than solely cultural practice.

Chapter 3
The factors that shape different epidemics

Epidemic disease, and AIDS in particular, is a disease of the body – but it is the presenting symptom. The manifestations of AIDS, illness and death, reveal the fractures, stresses, and strains in a society. This chapter shows that while at the most proximate level the chance of HIV transmission may depend on biological determinants, there are other factors that need to be considered, in particular social and economic poverty and inequality.

The overview of global epidemiology in Chapter 1 showed a range of epidemics. In a few places prevalence has peaked and fallen; in others it has risen to unexpected levels and remains high. There are settings where all the factors that would facilitate HIV spread seem to be in place yet there is no epidemic. While biomedical factors are critical, it is ultimately behaviours that will determine the shape of the epidemic. These depend on social and environmental factors – the position people occupy in society, their economic status, and how they are perceived and value themselves. Where vulnerabilities converge, we see the most serious epidemics.

If we can explain existing epidemics, can we predict new ones? Where prevalence has fallen, can we understand what happened in order that it can be replicated elsewhere?

Infections and epidemics don't happen randomly. Some diseases are limited to certain geographical environments – for example, to catch malaria a person must be in a malarial area and bitten by a mosquito carrying the parasite. People must be exposed to the pathogen. Even then, for an infection to take hold, the immune system must be unable to resist the disease-causing organism. This is true of all infectious illnesses: we see it every year with the common cold, when most people are exposed to the virus, but some individuals manage to stave off infection while others fall sick. Thus an individual's immune status is important in determining whether or not they are infected and how severely they are affected.

Drivers of disease are mostly social and economic. For example, living in poorly ventilated, crowded rooms increases the risk of exposure to and of contracting TB. Being undernourished and/or lacking vitamins and micronutrients will increase susceptibility to a plethora of illnesses and means people are sicker for longer.

Disease, globally and nationally, flourishes where there is poverty. In the rich countries of the world, the greatest disease burden is found among the poorer populations: those who are ill-nourished, poorly housed, and less well educated. With regard to nations, broadly speaking it is in the poorer ones where disease is more likely to thrive. Critical factors that can mitigate against poverty are social services and public health. Thus Cuba, or Kerala state in India, have healthier populations than their richer more inequitable neighbours.

On occasion there is a convergence of vulnerability that results in epidemic outbreaks. For example, prior to 1991, cholera had not been seen in the Americas for 100 years. In that year an outbreak began in Peru, after a ship in Lima harbour pumped its bilges of water that was contaminated by the *Vibrio cholerae* bacteria. The disease took hold in the city's slums, and then spread from slum

to slum across the Americas. Obviously ships had dischar~~ged~~
contaminated water before, both in Lima and other port~~s~~
However, in 1991 the slums had grown rapidly, the inha~~l~~
were the victims of a decade of economic crisis which resulted
in falling incomes and increased inequality. People were poorly
nourished and lacked access to basic infrastructure including
water, sanitation, and health services. The result was a regional
cholera epidemic.

Biomedical drivers

In order for a person to become infected, they must be in contact
with HIV with sufficient exposure for the infection to take
hold. Once contact has occurred, biomedical factors are the key
determinant of whether or not a person will be infected.

The most important biological influences are the virus sub-type
and the genetic make-up of those exposed. Some sub-types are
believed to be more infectious than others. This may be partly
why Southern Africa, where sub-type clade C is found, has such a
serious epidemic. The genetics may be important, operating at the
individual or population level, making some individuals or groups
more or less susceptible. This is controversial, as it is sometimes
interpreted as a form of 'genetic determinism' instead of the
natural 'reality' that results from the diversity of humankind.
Evolution is not 'kind' or 'cruel', although we may wish to construe
it as such. The importance of the virus type and genetics are areas
of continuing scientific research.

The stage of infection is crucial. For several months after
infection, there is an intense battle between the immune system
and the virus. During this period, the semen, vaginal fluids,
and blood contain many virus particles, increasing the chance
of infection for sexual partners and people who share injecting
equipment. There is then a period when the body rallies and the

al load is low. As the infection progresses, it will slowly climb and the CD4 cell count will fall, as shown in Figure 5 of the previous chapter.

Once the epidemic gains a hold in a society, it has a built-in momentum. The more people with early-stage infection, the greater the chance of someone having sex with such a person and being infected, so that a vicious cycle develops.

The virus has to breach the natural defences of the body, the skin or mucous membranes. Risk is higher for women as semen remains in the vagina after unprotected intercourse. This partly accounts for the greater number of women infected in heterosexually driven epidemics. The danger is increased by tearing in the vagina, which may occur during abusive sex or rape, especially in younger women whose vaginas are not mature, and thus interventions that delay sexual debut reduce transmission. Condoms provide a barrier, but are not female-controlled.

Sexually transmitted infections (STIs) are an important biological co-factor. Those that cause genital ulcers such as herpes, chancroid, and syphilis create a portal for the virus to enter the body, and at the same time the presence of the cells HIV seeks to infect, CD4 cells and macrophages, is increased. In a person with an STI, the number of virus particles released into blood, semen, and other body fluids increases, even if the infection is asymptomatic. An HIV-infected person is more likely to be infected by STIs and the severity and duration of these infections will be increased.

After sexual transmission, the next most important route of HIV infection is mother-to-child transmission (MTCT) with infants exposed through birth or breast-feeding. The viral load of the mother influences the probability of infection of the infant – the higher the load, the higher the risk. However, if a women has advanced disease, the chance of falling pregnant and carrying a child to term is decreased.

Other biomedical drivers include the use of unsafe blood and blood products and nosocomial (hospital-acquired) infections. In India in 2001, of the risk/transmission categories listed by the National AIDS Control Organization, 4.1% of AIDS cases resulted from contaminated blood or blood products. The practice there of paying blood donors may result in contaminated blood being collected, paid donors being more likely to live on the margins of society and to be infected. In China, it was estimated in 2002 that 9.7% of HIV cases were transmitted through illegal and unsafe practices associated with blood plasma collection.

While 'nosocomial' usually means infections acquired in hospital, with regard to HIV/AIDS it is taken to mean all infections transmitted in health care settings. If equipment is not adequately sterilized, then there is a danger of patient-to-patient transmission. Health workers are at risk through accidents involving body fluids such as needle stick injuries. All those caring for AIDS patients, including in the home, face some degree of danger and this rises if carers don't have adequate protective equipment such as gloves. Sharing drug-injecting equipment is an efficient way of spreading HIV, and this is the main driver in some settings.

One under-researched area is the effect of ill health from other causes on HIV transmission. There is evidence to suggest that any other infection will cause the viral load of HIV to rise rapidly and remain high for some time afterwards. For example, research shows that when an HIV-positive person has malaria the amount of virus in the blood increases tenfold, and thus such a person will be more infectious to his or her sexual partners. They may not want to have sex while they are sick, but when they recover their sex drive will return and infectivity is still high. Research in Kisumu in Kenya estimated that 5% of adult HIV infections were linked to malaria, and conversely, HIV infection increases susceptibility to other diseases, the Kenyan research also suggesting 10% of malaria cases were due to HIV. An HIV-positive individual with any other infection is likely to be sicker for longer and may be more likely to die.

Whether or not a man is circumcised, a biomedical solution, is important, as was discussed in the previous chapter. The routine offering of circumcision for male infants delivered in health care settings makes sense, but will take 20 or more years to impact on HIV prevalence. Had this happened in 1985, we would be reaping the benefits today.

Behaviours

In order for biomedical factors to come into play, a person has to have sex, or share needles with someone who is infected. There are a range of behaviours that increase risk. The AIDS epidemic has taught us unexpected lessons about human sexuality. The frequency of sexual intercourse does not vary greatly from country to country. There are a wide and intriguing variety of sexual practices, most of which are harmless and many are considered 'normal'. The behaviours that facilitate the spread of HIV are complex and dynamic, but global data suggest it is common for people to have more than one partner in their lifetime.

If someone does not have sex or sticks to one uninfected partner, then that person won't be sexually exposed to HIV (or any other sexually transmitted infection) provided their partner is also faithful. This applies in all sexual relationships – hetero- or homosexual. In societies where polygamy is practised, then as long as all parties are faithful, the same protections apply. Early AIDS prevention posters which, in most countries, said unequivocally 'Stick To One Partner' had to be adapted for Swaziland where polyandry is accepted and the king also has many wives – here, the posters had the less than catchy message: 'Be Faithful in Your Polygamous Family'.

Key behavioural factors are the age of sexual debut, sexual practices, number of partners, frequency of partner exchange, concurrency of partners, and mixing patterns including intergenerational sex. The younger a woman begins penetrative sex, the greater her risk of infection due to the danger of tearing of the vagina. The age of sexual debut is determined by her behaviour and those of her partners, and is influenced by social norms. Globally, data suggest that females have sex earlier than men, but trends for age at first sex are not clear. A meta-analysis of global sexual behaviour concluded trends towards earlier sexual experience are less pronounced than supposed. In developing countries, sexual activity is happening later, but prevalence of premarital sex increases if marriage is postponed. The data show the median age for first sexual intercourse for males was 16.5 in Kenya, Zambia, Brazil, Peru, and Britain. In the USA, it was 17.3. The oldest was 24.5, in Indonesia. For women, median age at first intercourse was lowest in a number of African countries: 15.5 in Ethiopia, Mozambique, Côte d'Ivoire, and Cameroon; the oldest was 20.5 in Rwanda. In the UK and USA, it was 17.5.

Data on sex and sexuality

We are all intrigued by sex and sexual behaviours, but collecting this information is complex. The first major study was by Dr Alfred Kinsey of Indiana University. The Kinsey Reports comprise two books on human sexual behaviour: *Sexual Behavior in the Human Male* (1948) and *Sexual Behavior in the Human Female* (1953). When released, this research was controversial, not just for the subject matter, but because it challenged many beliefs about sexuality, including the ideas that heterosexuality, faithfulness, and abstinence were ethical and statistical norms.

A basic problem with sexual behaviour data is that they are self-reported. This means that the data are subject to bias.

Most commonly, men over-report and women under-report partnerships and frequency of intercourse. This was well described in the title of an article on sexuality in Tanzania: *Secretive Females or Swaggering Males?* The meta-analysis published in *The Lancet* in 2006 shows how little data there are on sexual behaviour, and even less longitudinal information. One source of data is the Durex Global Sex Survey carried out annually since 1996. In 2005, it looked at 41 countries. It is web-based so has huge biases, but gives comparative and longitudinal data.

The question of sexual practices receives more salacious press than is deserved, although it is the area about which we know least. As far as HIV is concerned, some potentially harmful practices are widow inheritance, when a woman is 'inherited' by her deceased husband's brother, and the practice of 'dry sex', the use of herbs or other agents to dry out the vagina, which some believe increases (the man's) pleasure during sex, but the range of practices is immense. It is necessary to be open-minded, identify those that increase risk, understand how they do this, and find out what can be done about them.

The number of sexual partners *per se* seems less important. Men in Thailand (where the adult infection rate is 1.4%) and Rio de Janeiro (adult infection rate in Brazil is 0.5%) were more likely to report five or more casual partners in the previous year than men in Tanzania, Kenya, and Lesotho (where adult infection rates were 6.5%, 6.1%, and 23.2 % respectively). Adult prevalence in Zambia is 17%, but the 2005 Zambian Study found that over 97% of married women and 90% of married men indicated they had no non-marital partners in the previous year. The same survey found 26% of non-married people reported one 'non-regular partner' but only 4% reported two or three.

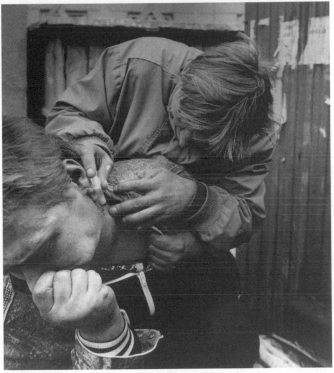

6. Needle-sharing, a high-risk behaviour

People in industrialized countries do not have significantly more or fewer partners in a lifetime, but their tendency is for serial monogamy. This means that they enter relationships which are maintained for months or years. The relationships involve a degree of commitment, and may be legally recognized as marriage or civil union. Serial monogamy traps the virus within a single relationship and so is not high risk for HIV transmission. The danger of infection increases when people have 'non-regular' partners or affairs.

While frequent partner change is hazardous, it is not common anywhere. The greatest risk is concurrency of partnering, when people have more than one partner and the relationships overlap for months or years. Writing in *The Lancet* in 2004, Halperin and Epstein noted that because infectivity is higher during the weeks and months after infection, concurrent partnering greatly exacerbates the spread of HIV and may be one of the main drivers. When a person in a network of concurrent relationships becomes infected, everyone is at risk. Mathematical models comparing serial monogamy and long-term concurrency showed that, in the latter, HIV transmission would be more rapid and the epidemic ten times greater.

Commercial sex, whether heterosexual and homosexual transactions, is potentially risky both for sex workers and their clients. In many settings, in the early years of the epidemic commercial sex workers were 'core transmitters'. A modelling exercise in Nairobi illustrated this. It assumed that 80% of sex workers were infected and had four clients per day, and 10% of men were infected and had four sexual partners per year. If women sex workers increased their clients' condom use from 10% to 80%, that was estimated to prevent 10,200 new infections. Increasing condom use among the men to 80% would avert only 88 infections. In Thailand, the early epidemic was spread by sex workers, but the '100% condom campaign', making condom use in brothels mandatory, was effective at bringing HIV spread under control. In Durban, research in the early 1990s found brothel-based sex workers (who used condoms) had negligible HIV infection.

Mixing patterns make it possible for an infection to be carried from one part of a country to another, across national borders, or to be introduced into previously closed circles. Here paths for transmission include both sex and drug use. For example, an oil worker who becomes infected in, say, Nigeria can carry the disease to his home country, then to, say, Indonesia in a matter of days.

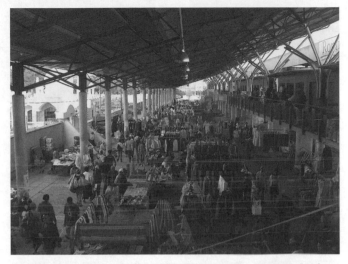

7. Warwick Junction in Durban, South Africa: where thousands of street traders serve many more thousands of daily commuters, and where HIV infection is high

A central Asian drug user can fly to any European capital in hours. With such mixing there is also the danger of re-infection and of new strains being created.

Mixing not only takes place across geographic regions but across age groups. Intergenerational sex, usually where men have younger female partners, is common in many societies. In countries where there is a heterosexual epidemic, the pattern is for women in their teens and twenties to have much higher prevalence than their male contemporaries. This is because they are having sex with older infected men, and sometimes this is transactional – for money, food, transport, and school or university fees.

The use of condoms is also a 'behaviour'. Correct, consistent condom use reduces the chances of HIV infection. When condoms were used in risky settings – among young people in Europe and the USA, and in brothels in Thailand – they prevented HIV spread or turned the epidemic around, but it is difficult to achieve consistent use other than in commercial and casual sexual encounters, and women may not have the power to insist their partners use condoms.

Social, economic, political, and other determinants

How people behave may determine their risk of infection, but behaviours result from the environment in which people live and operate. This milieu is, in turn, a function of local, national, and international factors; economics, politics, and culture. These are complex and varied and how we view them depends on our own values, backgrounds, and disciplines. The way the epidemic is influenced by these determinants is best illustrated by examples.

In Southern Africa, development of the mines and industry required a large workforce. The dominance of capitalism meant wages were tightly controlled. The colonial history and, in South Africa, subsequent apartheid legislation resulted in black labour being most exploited. Apartheid imposed strict controls on where black people could live and work and meant many South Africans were classified as migrants, effectively foreigners in their own country. Huge numbers of men travelled to work in the mines, factories, and on the farms. Foreign migrant miners were drawn primarily from Malawi, Lesotho, Botswana, Swaziland, Mozambique, and Namibia, and in the 1970s there were close to half a million foreigners employed on contracts in South Africa. In 1985 nearly two million black South Africans were classified as migrants. These people lived apart from their families, in hostel accommodation, and had to return home between contracts.

The effects of this dislocation and disempowerment have been well documented. When people are placed in circumstances in which they cannot maintain stable relationships, life is risky and pleasures are few and necessarily cheap, then sexually transmitted diseases will be rampant. This was true for all migrants. For migrant miners, their work was particularly dangerous, their control over most aspects of their lives was minimal, and they were disempowered in many respects. However, they had regular incomes. When gender inequality and the extreme poverty in the surrounding communities is considered, an ideal setting had been created for the spread of sexually transmitted infections.

During the 1980s, four large surveys were carried out to establish if HIV was present in South African populations outside of known high-risk groups. HIV was found by only one survey. The few cases were Malawian miners. Migration to and within South Africa created the perfect environment for the spread of HIV, not only in labour centres but in the migrants' home communities. The fracturing of families, changing gender dynamics, and increased poverty were major causes of the high levels of HIV.

Similar stories can be told of former communist countries. The collapse of communism was not good news for millions of citizens of the Soviet Union and Eastern Bloc. The system had provided many benefits, citizens were assured of employment, education, housing, health care, and even holidays; basic needs, and more, were met. The collapse of these economies has also been well documented. In the Ukraine, the per capita GDP (in purchasing power parity) fell from US\$ 6,372 in 1990 to a low of US\$ 3,194 in 1998. In 1994 alone, GDP declined by 22.9%. From having full employment, by 2000 the number of unemployed had reached close to three million, 12% of the economically active population. The pattern of societal collapse is seen across the region. Alcohol abuse was always common, but intravenous drug use increased dramatically, especially among the dispossessed and lost youth. The epidemic here has been driven by drug use – but this in turn is the result of economic and social disintegration and the consequent blow to the morale, hopes, and dreams of the younger generation.

In China, the epidemic of HIV among people selling blood, described in Chapter 1, has its roots in the political economy of the country. The peasants from whom the blood was collected are among the poorest, and selling blood is a survival strategy. The collapse of state medicine and introduction of fees meant that a ready, and unregulated, market existed. Ultimately, embracing the globalized economy will have partly driven China's epidemic.

Gender relations shape risk and behaviours. A woman's biology puts her at greater risk. Of crucial importance is the lack of power, and violence against women. Girls often feel pressured or forced into having sex. The Reproductive Health Research Unit Survey in South Africa reported that 28% of females and 16% of males aged 15 to 24 either 'did not want' or 'really did not want' their first sex. In Zambia, the Sexual Behaviour Survey in 2005 found 15.1% of females reported they were forced to have sex, and in 67.5% of cases it was by their husbands/boyfriends.

Some customs encourage early marriage and pregnancy; the marriage of young women to older men; and unequal partnering. These accept male dominance and female subservience. Globally, social norms emphasize female chastity and turn a blind eye to male promiscuity. In most of the poorer world, women are economically dependent on men, and sex work is the most extreme manifestation of this. Enabling female control of reproductive health would help the response to HIV/AIDS.

The relationship between HIV/AIDS and poverty is complex, both at the individual and national level. Botswana is, by most standards, a wealthy country. With a per capita income of US$ 4,372 in 2003, it has the third highest income in sub-Saharan Africa; Senegal by contrast has an income of just US$ 634 per capita. The prevalence rates among adults aged 15 to 49 in these countries are 24.1% in Botswana and 0.9% in Senegal. It would seem that simply being poor does not determine a country's HIV prevalence; rather, what is crucial is societal equality.

At the individual level, data are also less than straightforward. Demographic Health Survey (DHS) data from Burkina Faso, Cameroon, Ghana, Kenya, Lesotho, Malawi, Tanzania, and Uganda show that, contrary to evidence for other infectious diseases and intuitive expectations, HIV prevalence is not disproportionately higher among poorer adults in sub-Saharan Africa. Indeed in all countries, except Ghana, the trend is the wealthier the person, the more likely they are to be HIV positive. When confounding and mediating factors (such as mobility and urban residence) are controlled for, wealthier adults are at least as likely to be HIV-infected as poorer ones. This is particularly marked for women. In Kenya, 3.9% of the poorest quintile of women were infected; for the richest, it was 12.2%; for men, these figures were 3.4% and 7.3% respectively.

Conclusion

While, at the most proximate level, the chance of HIV transmission may depend on biological determinants, they are only a part of the picture. Developing drugs, vaccines, and microbicides, circumcising men, and putting people on treatment are technical and biomedical responses. Unfortunately, this disease does not lend itself to simple technical solutions.

The real challenge is to change behaviours to reduce risk. Behaviours can be modified, and the evidence suggests that there are a few key interventions that would have a significant impact on the progress of the epidemic. These include reducing concurrent partnering and delaying sexual debut for young women. Beyond this are the messages that have been used since the early days of the epidemic: abstinence, fidelity, and condom use.

Both behaviours and biomedical factors are determined by how a society operates at the macro level: the culture, politics, and economics. These factors are crucial, and most important are gender relations and income equality. The central issue is how people treat and see one another. A society in which people respect the views and choices of others is one in which unsafe sex is less likely to occur.

Preventing HIV transmission requires a greater understanding of the determinants of the epidemic. Unfortunately for the 40 million people currently infected, the 20+ million who have died, and their families and communities, prevention has not worked. We need to understand how AIDS and its impact will work its way through society. This is the theme of the following chapters.

Chapter 4
Illness, deaths, and populations

This chapter looks at what AIDS is doing to populations through demographic indicators. HIV-infected people experience episodes of illness that lead to death. All effects flow from these illnesses and deaths. Although these indicators are important, and are being dramatically altered in some settings, they have their limitations and these too are discussed.

Demography is the study of population dynamics, which collects data on quantifiable events and uses this for analysis and projections. The basic data sources are censuses, ideally done every ten years, collecting a range of information on numbers of people, households, age, gender, education, employment, and religion. Between censuses population is tracked through registration, particularly of births and deaths. Demographers want to know, at a minimum, how many children are born, the fertility rate, death rate, and migration. Data collection may be problematic, especially in poorer countries where censuses are infrequent and it often takes several years for analysis and release of data. Smaller household surveys and the Demographic and Health Surveys referred to earlier provide additional and useful information. The lack of data is a constraint in understanding both current and future effects of AIDS.

The demographic consequences of AIDS are increased deaths, especially among those aged 20 to 49; rising infant and child mortality; falling life expectancy; changes in the population size, growth, and structure; and a growth in the numbers of orphans. How serious these impacts are will depend on the location, size, and age of the epidemic and the underlying demographics of a country. For example, in the USA, prior to ART, AIDS was the leading cause of mortality among young men. In Southern Africa, prevalence rates rose rapidly from 1992, but it was only in the early part of the 21st century that there was a measurable and significant rise in the number of illnesses and deaths, and this is still growing. The number of deaths in Uganda peaked in the 1990s but the country is dealing with one million orphans. Shrinking birth rates in Eastern Europe mean relatively small epidemics have disproportionate impacts here.

Although it is difficult to look far into the future, we can make predictions. In most countries we have a reasonably clear idea of the magnitude of the HIV epidemic (within a range). Even very resource-poor countries are able to predict illnesses and deaths, and in many countries this was done as part of planning for ART roll-out. We can predict demographic impacts and be realistically sure of what they will look like for ten years, and we can factor in treatment and develop scenarios.

At the root of the difficulties in understanding the effects of the epidemic are what we measure, and when and how we measure it. Demography looks at events: an AIDS death is an event. The proceeding period of illness, prolonged and debilitating for the individual, and costly and demoralizing for families, households, and communities, is part of a process and is not measured by demographers. Many impacts are felt after death, and there is evidence that AIDS deaths have more serious consequences for survivors than deaths from other causes. Most 'post-death' consequences are not measured by demography.

Increased mortality

Increased deaths in younger adults are the most measurable effect of AIDS. This has been dramatically illustrated by data from South Africa, which has one of the best vital registration systems in the poor world. In 2001 the Medical Research Council released a report analysing the registered deaths reported to the Department of Home Affairs. This report was controversial but its findings were unequivocal. It showed the pattern of mortality had shifted from the old to the young, particularly to young women; there was differential mortality between men and women, which fitted with the pattern projected by AIDS models, and it concluded that the future burden of the epidemic was broadly predictable.

This changing mortality, with the most recent data, is shown in Figure 8. In 1997 the highest number of female deaths was in the 70 to 79 age group. Deaths among younger women increased until, by 2000, this figure was highest for women in their late 20s and early 30s, and continuing to rise. Among men the peak in 'new' mortality is slightly later, but with the same dramatic change in the pattern and number of deaths.

The cause of death is not ascribed: the graphs show only recorded numbers of deaths. This increased mortality simply should not be happening, especially in post-apartheid South Africa. Government policy, since the transition, has been to improve the lives of all, especially the poor and women. Health services have been expanded and are free to pregnant women and children. Water, sanitation, power, and housing are being provided; and there are a range of social grants available. South Africans, especially women, should be living longer and better lives. These graphs should sound a clarion call of warning as they show the effects of a devastating AIDS epidemic; instead they are ignored or explained away.

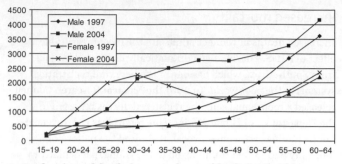

8. **Total registered deaths by age and year of death, South Africa**

The pattern of mortality shown in Figure 8 is found across high-prevalence countries, and has severe consequences for society. Those who die have received whatever education and training is available; many will be in the middle ranks of employment, gaining experience and skills. This is also when most people have had children.

Treatment not only reduces mortality but allows people to resume normal lives. Significant numbers of people need to access treatment before the figures at the population level will reflect gains. In 2002 the Actuarial Society of South Africa (ASSA) suggested that the national ART programme would only reduce the number of deaths from 495,000 to 381,000 per annum in 2010.

Infant and child mortality rises for two reasons. Firstly, children born to infected mothers have, in the absence of intervention, about a 30% chance of being infected. Prevention of mother-to-child transmission greatly reduces this, but those who are infected have poor life expectancy. About 25% of HIV-infected babies develop symptoms of AIDS or die within the first year. In the developed world, 70% of those infected at birth are alive at 6 years and 50% at 9 years, but in the poor world progression rates are faster. Treating children is a growing global priority.

Demographics: key measures

Life expectancy is a single index describing the level of mortality in a given population at a particular time as measured in years of life. It is the age at which a person can expect to die. Currently, according to UNDP's 2006 report, Japan has the longest life expectancy at 82 years; the lowest is Swaziland at just 31.3 years.

Infant mortality measures the number of children dying before age 1 per 1,000 live births. The lowest is 2, in Iceland; the highest is Sierra Leone's 166. Child mortality measures the number of deaths in children under 5 per 1,000 live births and is therefore a better measure of the impact of AIDS. Sierra Leone has the highest child mortality at 283; the lowest is 3 in Singapore and Iceland (it is 6 in the UK and 8 in the USA). Reducing child mortality by two-thirds is a Millennium Development Goal.

Other important measures are the crude birth rate (CBR) and crude death rate (CDR) and the total fertility rate (TFR). The CBR and CDR are the total number of births and deaths respectively per 1,000 people per year. The TFR is the number of live births per woman in her reproductive life.

The dependency ratio is the ratio of the economically dependent part of the population (those too young or too old to work) to those who are productive. Generally, individuals under the age of 15 and over the age of 65 are considered to be dependent. The dependency ratio is given as a rate per 100.

The sex ratio is the number of males to females. At birth, it is usually 105 males to 100 females, though higher male mortality means there are more females than males among the elderly: in Germany, 70 men for every 100 women over 65.

The second reason for increased child deaths is mortality among infected mothers. Losing a mother for any reason has an adverse impact on child survival. A 2004 review of the demographic and socio-economic impact of AIDS, published by the journal *AIDS*, noted the death of a mother increased the chance of a child dying by three times in the year before the mother's death and five times in the year after the death. Increased child mortality was not affected by the mother's cause of death, but HIV-infected mothers are much more likely to die.

The most detailed projections of the likely effects of AIDS come from the US Bureau of the Census. Their 2004 report, *The AIDS Pandemic in the 21st Century*, produced country data 'with AIDS' and 'without AIDS'. The figures are sobering.

In Botswana, in 2002 the crude death rate was estimated at 28.6 per 1,000, without AIDS it would have been a mere 4.8: by 2010, it may be as high as 42.8. For Tanzania, the 2002 figures are: without AIDS 12.1, with AIDS 17.3. Because Tanzania's epidemic is more advanced, by 2010 the CDR may have fallen slightly to 17.1. In Guyana, the death rate in 2002 was 8.9, 2.3 above what it would have been without AIDS, and by 2010 it may be 13.2. The greatest increase in Asia is projected for Myanmar at 2.2 deaths per 1,000 above the non-AIDS level in 2010. For child mortality rates, the greatest increase is in Botswana: in 2002, the rate was estimated at 107.1, without AIDS it would have been only 30.6; by 2010, it is projected to be 122.9 instead of falling to 22.8. In Cambodia, AIDS is adding 7 deaths per 1,000 to child mortality, and in Haiti 10.5 deaths.

Falling life expectancy

Demographers and international policy-makers agree that AIDS is knocking years off life expectancy, especially in Africa. In 2003, the UN Population Division looked at the impact of AIDS on 38 African, 5 Asian, 8 Latin American and Caribbean countries, the

Russian Federation, and the USA. Data are not presented for individual countries, probably a 'political' decision as governments react adversely to being named when the news is bad. The data in Table 4 show that the impact of AIDS will amplify and be felt most strongly from 2010 to 2015. A sustained and expanded roll-out of treatment could change this.

The Bureau of the Census produced projections for individual countries. The impacts are expected to be dramatic. By 2010, life expectancy could be just 26.7 years in Botswana and 27.1 years in Mozambique. Access to therapy by sufficient numbers of people could change this. Worst affected outside Africa are Guyana, which is predicted to lose 14.3 years of life, and Cambodia, which will lose 4.2 years. The data don't show what this catastrophic decline in life expectancy will actually mean for these societies. Will it affect societal ability to function? This issue is returned to in later chapters, but it is worth stressing we don't know, because we have yet to experience such impacts and demographers do not think in terms of what these predictions mean for society at large.

Changing population composition, growth, and dependency ratios

Increased numbers of deaths reduce population size. Some 2.8 million people, mostly young adults, are dying from AIDS every year. In the worst affected countries the mortality is considerable: UNAIDS estimates that in 2005 South Africa had 320,000 deaths from AIDS, Nigeria 220,000, and Zimbabwe 180,000. The deaths are cumulative: by 2015, some 6 million South Africans may have died of AIDS – 13% of the population.

Population growth decreases through premature deaths; a reduction in fertility; and changing sexual behaviours. As the epidemic progresses there are fewer women of child-bearing age. HIV-positive women are less likely to conceive and carry the infant to term, thus further reducing the number of live births.

Table 4. Estimated and projected impact of HIV/AIDS on mortality indicators

Life expectancy at birth (years)	All 53 countries			38 African countries			7 countries with prevalence of 20% or more		
	1995–2000	2010–2015	2020–2025	1995–2000	2010–2015	2020–2025	1995–2000	2010–2015	2020–2025
Without AIDS	63.9	68.4	70.8	52.7	58.3	62.1	62.3	67.0	69.6
With AIDS	62.4	64.2	65.9	47.0	47.1	51.3	50.2	37.6	41.0
Absolute difference	1.5	4.1	4.9	5.7	11.3	10.8	12.0	29.4	28.6
Percentage difference	2.4	6.1	6.9	10.9	19.3	17.4	19.3	43.9	41.1

The potential effects of behaviour change are considerable. Condoms may be used to protect against disease, but also have an impact on fertility. An increased age of sexual debut will reduce the total fertility rate.

In most countries, AIDS simply means the population will grow more slowly. In Thailand, growth is expected to be 1% per annum rather than 1.1%; in India and China, the impact will be negligible as the populations are so large and the epidemic is, relatively, so small. In other countries, AIDS will greatly reduce population growth. The Bureau of the Census estimated Botswana's growth rate in 2002 was –0.2% per annum instead of 2.3%, and by 2010 it will be –2.1%. In South Africa, the growth rate is projected to be –1.4%, in Swaziland –0.4%, and in Lesotho and Mozambique –0.2%. Without AIDS these populations would be growing. The impact of this on the national psyche, economy, and social welfare system will be considerable. As yet there is no evidence that the impact is being thought through, and is an area requiring more research.

In Latin America and the Caribbean, the Bahamas and Guyana will see the greatest relative impact, with growth rates reduced from 1% to 0.5%. In Eastern Europe, the impact of AIDS will exacerbate an already troubling demographic situation, where there are very low total fertility rates and populations are declining. By 2030, the median age of the Russian population will be over 40, with half the population having been born before 2000. By 2015, there will be just four workers for every three non-workers, with a dramatic shift among the non-working-age population toward the elderly. AIDS is increasing mortality among the current 15- to 30-year-old age group, so that there will be fewer working-age people at a time when they are sorely needed.

As Figure 3 showed, peak mortality is between 25 and 35 for women, and 30 and 45 for men. This alters the population

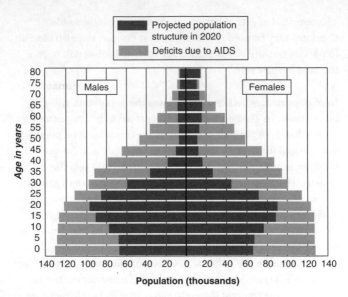

9. Altered population structure due to HIV/AIDS, Botswana

structure and dependency ratios. An extreme change in population structure is shown in Figure 9 – a projected population pyramid for Botswana in 2020. The outer bars show the shape and size of the population in the absence of AIDS, the inner bars show what it could be. By 2020, instead of just under 60,000 women in the 40 to 50 age group there will be about 12,000. There will be half the children under 5 that there would have been in the absence of AIDS. While the gaps in the under-25 age group are a combination of mortality and births that did not occur, among the over-25 age group the changing pyramid is due to deaths.

The dependency rate will increase, placing demands on the government and society to provide education for the young, and health and social support care for both the young and the elderly. It adversely affects economic growth by depressing the national savings rate and reducing future domestic resources available for investment. The dependency rate in Zambia is 99 dependants for every 100 adults, in Uganda it is 112. An excellent example of the potential benefits of changing dependency comes from Ireland, where in 1970 the TFR was 3.9, but by 2006 it was estimated to have fallen to 1.86. The dramatic and sustained economic growth in Ireland, described as a 'Celtic Tiger', was in part due to the availability of resources which had previously been tied up in educating and supporting the large number of young people. Of course, ageing populations cause problems but these are different.

Conventional dependency ratio calculations assume most adults are productive, but in generalized AIDS epidemics a significant number are chronically sick and properly belong in the 'dependants' category, a factor that needs to be considered. There will also be changes in the gender balance. In heterosexually driven epidemics more women will die than men at younger ages. Over the next 20 years, in many countries, men between the ages of 35 and 54 will outnumber women. This may motivate men to seek sexual relationships with younger and younger women, increasing HIV infection rates, and leading to a vicious cycle of transmission operating for generations. The changing gender and age structure of populations and the consequences desperately need thought and research. As the epidemic bites, families are being held together by the elderly, especially the grandmothers.

Orphaning

As conventionally understood, an orphan is a child who has lost both parents, but the definition has changed, in large part due to AIDS. The current definition used by UNICEF, other international agencies, and most NGOs is that an orphan is a child under the age of 18 who has lost one or both parents. Maternal orphans have lost a mother, paternal orphans a father, and double orphans both parents.

Globally, orphan numbers were declining, and despite the AIDS epidemic this trend has been sustained in Asia, Latin America, and the Caribbean. However, in sub-Saharan Africa numbers of orphans have grown dramatically. AIDS orphans increased in number from fewer than one million in 1990 to 12 million in 2005. In 2003, 12.3% of all children in sub-Saharan Africa were orphans (in Asia it was 7.3% of children, and 6.2% in Latin America and the Caribbean).

Countries with high HIV prevalence levels or recent armed conflict have the most orphans. Botswana has the peak rate of orphaning in sub-Saharan Africa, with 20% of its children orphaned. South Africa has the largest total number, an estimated 1.2 million AIDS orphans. Beyond Africa, the highest level of orphaning is in Haiti, where 15% of children are in this situation.

The number of orphans will increase. UNICEF estimates that by 2010, globally, there will be 142 million orphans, of whom 50 million will be in sub-Saharan Africa, and here 18.4 million or 36.8% will be due to AIDS. There is no estimate of AIDS orphaning in the other regions. Ugandan data show orphaning peaks some 15 years after prevalence, which means that in many countries we will not see the crest of the orphan wave until after 2020.

There are limits to what demography shows us. Children orphaned by AIDS have different experiences and bear additional burdens to those orphaned by other causes. The death of a parent is preceded by prolonged illness. If one parent is infected, there is a probability that the other parent is infected and both will die: double orphans are more disadvantaged than single orphans. When orphans are taken in by grandparents (usually grandmothers), they face the prospect of losing elderly caregivers too, effectively a repeat orphaning. Research gives us numbers, but the psychological impact is still to be assessed.

Chapter 5
The impact of AIDS on production and people

This chapter discusses the effects of the epidemic on economies, production, and social reproduction. AIDS does not, at the macroeconomic level, appear to have a significant and measurable impact. However, long-term economic growth and development depends on investment in people, and human capital is particularly threatened. As the level of focus narrows to the community, households, and families, HIV/AIDS has clear and measurable effects, which are worse for women. Of particular importance are the adverse consequences on subsistence agriculture, especially since there are other stressors at work.

Tracking the social and economic costs of AIDS is more complex than measuring the demographic consequences but the reasons are similar. The epidemic does not have a long history but what we measure is what has happened, not what will happen. Then there is the danger of research which may not ask the right questions or look in the right places. Most surveys look at households, but AIDS means some disappear. There is tension between intensive ethnographic research done at an individual level, and national survey instruments that lose detail.

People, communities, and economies have coping strategies, and the presence of AIDS means adaptations occur. Some predictions of what AIDS would do were simply wrong. An example was the forecast of 'feral bands of AIDS orphans roaming the streets and engaging in criminal activity': this has not happened. However, most illnesses and deaths are still to come. Unlike demographers who are able to model and project, it seems social scientists, policy-makers, and politicians do not have the tools, skills, or even the wish to look into the future.

The conundrum of macroeconomic effects

Trying to ascribe causality to HIV/AIDS for economic impact is problematic, as there are so many other factors to be considered, from the price of oil to national fiscal policy. Conventional economics misses the complexity and full significance of the epidemic. AIDS cannot be treated as an 'exogenous' influence that can be 'tacked on'. In many settings AIDS is a reality, there is no 'without AIDS' scenario.

The models produced by economists in the early 1990s predicted a negative relationship between HIV/AIDS and growth. World Bank economists estimated a 1.2% point reduction in annual growth for a 20% prevalence rate. However, AIDS does not appear to have held back economic growth in Uganda, Botswana, or South Africa. Uganda, with the worst epidemic in the world at the beginning of the 1990s, managed consistent economic growth, estimated at 6.5% per annum from 1991 to 2002. Botswana's growth rate over the same period was 5.6%. South Africa posted its 47th month of consecutive growth in March 2006, and growth was estimated at 4.4%. Why do the models of HIV/AIDS impact and the data appear at odds? Might these countries have grown faster in the absence of AIDS? It is possible that the epidemic may be contributing to Malawi's miserable economic performance or Zimbabwe's collapse, but this is difficult to assess.

Economic theory states growth is determined by capital accumulation (both physical and human) and total factor productivity. HIV/AIDS is assumed to affect growth through reduced savings and investment, and by reducing the size of the labour force, which lowers efficiency and productivity. Capital accumulation, physical or human, is a central tenet of most growth theories. The Asian economic successes were due in part to high levels of capital accumulation driven by domestic savings.

Physical capital accumulation happens through savings and investment. HIV/AIDS affects this at the individual, firm, and international level. For instance, families affected by HIV/AIDS may deplete their savings and assets in order to cope with increased expenditure and income shocks. Similarly, firm profits (and hence saving and investment) may decrease due to lower labour productivity and increased AIDS-related expenditure. Falls in life expectancy and increased mortality shorten planning horizons and lower incentives to save and invest.

Does AIDS affect investment flows at the international and national level? Assessing a lack of capital flows requires measuring something that has not happened, which is nigh on impossible. There are a few recorded instances of HIV/AIDS deterring investors. The Swazi press reported that a Taiwanese textile firm had decided to start its factory employing 5,000 workers in Lesotho due to high HIV prevalence in Swaziland. The investors did not want to train workers who, they believed, would soon fall ill and die.

There is also the vexing question of per capita income. This is calculated by dividing the total output of the country by the number of people, usually expressed in US dollars and adjusted for what the dollars will buy in the country: the purchasing power parity. Thus the per capita income in Luxembourg, the world's richest country, is over US$ 62,000, while the poorest, Sierra Leone, is US$ 548. The per capita income in the UK and USA is US$ 27,147 and US$ 37,562 respectively. If the people who die are contributing little and their deaths do not affect overall production, then in *economic terms* the per capita income may go up. This economic reality is uncomfortable and rarely talked about as it values lives differently.

Thus, if the epidemic is located among the poor or in very poor countries, the impact may be minimal. Where peasant farmers' contribution to the formal economy is insignificant and they expect little from the state, then their disappearance may be *economically* insignificant. In a society with high unemployment among the unskilled, losing these people will not have the same *economic* impact as when there is a skills shortage and the loss is among the skilled.

So what are we to conclude about the macroeconomic impact of this disease? Theory suggests that AIDS will cause economies to grow more slowly. There is, as yet, little clear evidence of this. The two key phrases are 'as yet' and 'little clear evidence'. In many cases, the effects are still to be felt and depend not only on numbers, but also the location and context. In Eastern Europe, although numbers are not large, infections are occurring in a context of declining populations and poor health, therefore AIDS may well affect the economies. The other part of the deconstruction of 'as yet' is that economies are highly dynamic and will adapt. For example, if certain skills become in short supply then the response might be to buy in those skills or to mechanize.

AIDS and the private sector

The impact of AIDS on the private sector will depend on the scale of the epidemic in the country or area, the capital labour mix of the firm, the role of the government in terms of regulation and sharing the burden of AIDS, and what actions individual companies take to avert the effects of the epidemic.

In some countries, firms are experiencing increased illness and death among workers which results in rising costs and falling productivity. AIDS equates to a payroll tax. However, the 'tax' ranges from 0.5% of aggregate annual labour costs in a retail business in South Africa to 10.8% in tourism in Zambia, depending on HIV prevalence, the type of industry, and employee benefits.

More interesting is what decreased productivity costs companies. This is hard to measure except where workers are paid according to output. The first such study by Boston University's Center for International Health and Development (CIHD) looked at a tea plantation in Kenya where workers were paid per kilogram of leaf plucked. The CIHD research reviewed records of output and absenteeism from January 1997 to December 2002. HIV-infected individuals plucked on average 3.6 kg/day less tea 2 to 3 years prior to death, 5.1 kg/day less 1 year prior to death, and 9.3 kg/day less when approaching death. In the 3 years leading up to death, HIV-positive workers used between 3.4 and 11.0 more days of sick leave, depending on the stage of illness. Recent research with this cohort shows the benefits of ART. When workers were put on treatment, productivity increased to about 80% of that among uninfected workers.

Firms are not helpless in the face of the epidemic. They have a range of responses open to them – from changing the composition of the workforce, to reducing their benefits, to, in the most extreme cases, relocating to places with lower HIV prevalence. AIDS can be factored in like any other cost or threat.

Unknown is how the epidemic affects the environment in which companies operate. The impacts of HIV/AIDS, including decreasing productivity, are often exacerbated in the public sector when compared to the private sector. In the public sector, job security and benefits are a substitute for salary and there is limited capacity to respond. The costs of public-sector benefits are borne by government; the costs of declining efficiency are borne by society at large.

AIDS and human capital

In the 1950s, a bright future was predicted for African countries but people were pessimistic about Asia. However, from 1965 to 1998 the average annual growth rate was 7.5% in East Asia and the Pacific, and per capita incomes grew by 5.7%. In South Asia, growth was 4.9% and per capita incomes grew by 2.7%. The corresponding figures for sub-Saharan Africa were growth of 2.6% and a decline in per capita incomes of –0.3%.

Today, Asia maintains high growth and people have seen benefits in terms of human development. Poverty and child mortality have declined and life expectancy risen. Latin America has not seen the same economic growth, but there have been gains, particularly with regard to social service delivery and social development. Sub-Saharan Africa remains the laggard: poverty has increased, the number of people malnourished remains high, and life expectancy is falling.

The HIV/AIDS epidemic is making a bad situation worse, and may soon become one of the primary drivers of African under-development. Patterns of development have been different in Asia, Latin America, and Africa because of dissimilar investments in human capital, which was highest in Asia. AIDS means a growing inability to invest in human capital, including education and health, and growing numbers of orphans.

The role of the state is crucial. As early as the mid-1700s, the economist Adam Smith argued that the state should create the conditions in which the market could work, and this still holds true. The state needs, at a minimum, to ensure the rule of law, property rights, and accountability. In the early stages of development good economic governance is critical. If the converse is true and the market can't work due to poor human rights, instability, or corruption, then investment won't happen. AIDS has an impact on state capacity, to which we will return in the next chapter.

The second critical area is increased productivity which comes from investing in people. In many Asian countries, the state and parents poured resources into education. This, with the demographic transition – smaller families and a lower dependency ratio – created the environment in which investment was both possible and desirable.

Health in itself is an important goal. It is people's priority, as a survey for the 2000 Millennium Development Summit found. There are links between health and economic growth, as articulated in the WHO's 2001 Commission on Macroeconomics and Health, which noted health and education are cornerstones of human capital, and the basis of an individual's economic productivity. Every 10% improvement in life expectancy results in an annual rise in economic growth of 0.3 to 0.4 percentage points. The effects of falling life expectancies described in the previous chapter have not been considered by development agencies and economists.

The effect of AIDS on the next generation, the human capital of the future, is considerable. There are fewer children and more orphans. Orphaning is the measured event, but is part of a process, as illustrated in the text box overleaf. Priscilla's experience with AIDS began before her mother died. Priscilla nursed her mother and watched her die, a psychological trauma. She is parenting her younger sister while she is still attending school, which is clearly a struggle. The father does not make an appearance.

Education is crucial. Even in the absence of AIDS, children face barriers to school attendance. There has been a global push to abolish school fees. A survey presented at a DFID/UNICEF Global Partners Forum meeting in London in 2006 showed

The story of Priscilla in the Free State in South Africa

'I lost my mum six months ago, she was very sick. I did everything for her. Whenever she wanted water to drink I would get it for her. I would spoon-feed her and dress her.

When I had to go to school I had to ask my neighbours to look after her, and particularly the carers from the clinic. She was really ill for five months and did not have a doctor.

Before my mother was sick she did everything for me. She promised to take me to school to get a good education, which I'm worried about now. Whenever I look at the clothes my mum liked, they remind me of her.

When I wake up I wash myself and sometimes I eat breakfast if there's pap [cornmeal porridge] or bread. Then I go to school, which is far to walk to. I like playing netball and I love school very much, especially politics and history, and learning about things that took place around the world and here.

Every day I come home and wash my uniform. I wash my little sister and, if there is homework, I do this too. I cook pap for everyone, which takes a long time on the [Primus] stove. When my older sister comes, she eats in her bedroom with her children, and me and my younger sister eat together.

I want to finish school and raise my little sister in my mum's house. The house is registered in my name now.'

Missing Mothers, Save the Children UK (London, 2006), p. 4

that of 92 developing countries, 76 charged fees. But fees are not just charged by governments, they include levies by schools for textbooks and stationery; Parent-Teacher Association (PTA) charges; and the costs of compulsory uniforms. There are also indirect costs such as transport, and the forgone benefits of the labour the child would provide were they working.

It is harder for orphans to access education. Orphaning means there are fewer resources to enable the children to attend school, and orphans face psychological pressures and stigma. A teacher in KwaZulu-Natal reported, 'we can tell which children are orphans, they are dirty and uncared for and have many difficulties'. Priscilla at age 14 has taken on the task of getting her younger sister to school, a burden to both.

However, the numbers of child-headed households are not as high as predicted. Data from UNICEF and USAID-supported surveys in sub-Saharan Africa show that 9 out of 10 orphans are cared for by the extended family. This is commendable, but taking in additional children often means meagre resources have to stretch further. Siblings may be parted, which can be traumatic. In Zambia, in 2005, I heard the story of how a grandmother and her sister had taken in the two grandchildren, boys aged 9 and 13, when their mother died. Both had gone to homes with an income, care, and love, though one child was taken to the north, the Copperbelt, the other to Livingstone in the south. The women remarked the boys really missed each other and were overjoyed to see each other on the infrequent occasions they met.

Devastating agriculture systems: the 'new variant famine' hypothesis

There is evidence that AIDS is having an overwhelming effect on agriculture, primarily but not only through the impact on labour. The HIV/AIDS epidemic has such far-reaching adverse implications that it can be argued, in some settings, we are witnessing a 'new variant famine'. This was discussed in an article I co-authored with Alex de Waal, published in *The Lancet* in 2003.

This is best illustrated with examples from Southern Africa, which since the turn of the new century has been experiencing a large-scale food crisis. Proximate causes include drought, a lack of inputs such as seed and fertilizer, as well as mismanagement of national food stockpiles and distribution. The current profile of vulnerability to starvation is different from previous drought-induced famines and rural livelihoods are collapsing.

In Zambia's Central Province, the effect of adult illness and death on farm production was assessed among smallholder cotton farming households between 1999 and 2003. There were high levels of death and illness: 40% of households had an adult death in the study period, and 36% reported an adult was sick 'regularly'. This work showed that where households experienced the death of a previously healthy working-aged adult, the amount of land planted to maize declined by 16% and that under cotton by 11%. Across the border in a Zimbabwean communal farming area, a study found an adult death resulted in a 45% decline in

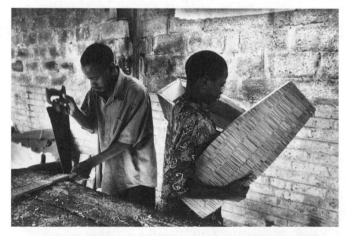

10. Ignacious Ngulu and Gibson Mufwayo at work building a child's coffin. They are members of the Kamitondo Youth Coffin-Making Cooperative in Kitwe, Zambia. More than 20% of pregnant women are HIV positive in this area, so in the absence of mother-to-child prevention programmes they are constantly called upon to supply coffins for children and babies who have died from AIDS-related infections

a household's marketed maize; where the cause of death was identified as AIDS, the loss was 61%.

Illness among subsistence farmers means high-value and nutritious crops, such as cereals and oilseeds, are replaced by ones that are easier to cultivate but are lower-value and less nutritious. The area under cultivation is reduced. There is an impact on animal husbandry, as livestock receive less attention. In Swaziland, both the quantity and the quality of the nation's cattleholding are diminishing.

AIDS is eroding the resilience of rural livelihoods, by undermining coping strategies. Food crisis coping strategies depend critically on labour availability, skill, and experience. The disease and impacts cluster at the household level and (to a lesser extent) within communities. Because AIDS changes age and gender distribution, there are fewer mature adults (especially women), and relatively more teenagers and people in their early 20s. The loss of older people means skills and knowledge are not passed on – 'institutional memory' is lost. Women are particularly important in time of famine as they often have knowledge of wild foods that can be gathered.

Agriculture, even of the most basic subsistence type, does not operate in a vacuum. AIDS means key services such as marketing cooperatives and agricultural extension are less efficient due to staff attrition and declining morale. In Malawi, attrition due to death among the Ministry of Agriculture and Industry staff rose from 0.45% to 1.1% annually between 1996 and 1998.

Malnutrition has adverse implications in high HIV-prevalence settings. Nutritional status is a determinant of risk of transmission both between adults and from mothers to infants, and undernourished people are more likely to be infected. Those who are infected endanger their health by going hungry, as HIV replicates more rapidly in malnourished individuals, hastening the progression from HIV to AIDS. People living with HIV have greater nutritional requirements. There is a vicious cycle, since some illnesses associated with HIV reduce appetite and even ability to eat, oral candidiasis being an example, and others such as diarrhoea inhibit the absorption of nutrients. In normal famines it is possible for adults to go for periods without food and survive, but this is not so with HIV.

The issue is not simply overall availability of food, but rather the ability of the poorest members of society to purchase it. This is especially the case in urban areas. Zimbabwe provides an extreme example. The Famine Early Warning Systems Network declared, in March 2006, that macroeconomic collapse had put the cost of basic foodstuffs beyond the reach of most Zimbabweans. Despite good rains, output of maize was well below requirements. The cost of imported maize grain in Harare in January 2006 was 1860% more than in January 2005, and the annual rate of inflation in May 2006 reached 1193%. In June 2006, the minimum wage in the commercial sector only covered 40% of the cost of the minimum food basket, and the economic collapse has continued.

A detailed case study of the desperately poor country of Malawi, co-edited by myself and Anne Conroy, Malcolm Blackie, Justin Malewezi, and Jeffrey Sachs, published in late 2006, paints a bleak picture. Nationally, HIV prevalence was estimated at 14.1% of adults. In the Central Region, a survey by Care International found a significant number of households suffered from chronic illness and were unable to provide the labour needed for even low-productivity subsistence agriculture. Between 22% and 64% of households in study sites suffered from chronic sickness, leading to loss of labour. In households with labour loss, 45% delayed agricultural operations, 23% left land fallow, and 26% changed the crop mix. Resources were being used for health care and funerals, and this led to even lower levels of household income and nutrition.

Female-headed households were worst affected. Malawian women do much of the agricultural work and combine this with child-bearing and -rearing and household responsibilities. They have the 'double burden of care', as they are most likely to suffer from HIV/AIDS and are also responsible for caring for others.

Before 2002, many Malawians were consuming fewer than 1,500 calories per day. Since then the country has faced a number of major food crises. The per capita income of Malawi is US\$ 605, life expectancy a mere 39.7 years, and two-thirds of the population live below the national poverty line. In such poverty, few households have assets: a household survey in the late 1990s found just over one-third of all households owned a bed and less than a half owned chairs and tables.

The picture that emerges from Malawi is of an increasingly malnourished, stressed society. There is long-term environmental degradation: 85% of energy comes from traditional fuel, mainly wood, leading to massive deforestation. Fish production from Lake Malawi has declined by nearly 40%, which is particularly significant since fish contributes 60–70% of the total animal protein consumption. Poor governance has been a persistent theme. The country is highly indebted and aid-dependent – in 2003 aid accounted for close to 30% of GDP. The economy is stagnant: the 2005 growth rate was only 1.9%. Where poverty is this deep, there is virtually no scope for normal coping mechanisms. AIDS may be the last straw; Malawi may yet provide an example of AIDS as a cause of state failure.

Malawi may be an extreme example, but across the world the pressure caused by AIDS needs to be seen in the context of other stressors. The most important one for subsistence farmers is climate change. As with AIDS, vulnerability to climate change is differentiated and it is the poor who are most exposed. In Africa, one manifestation of climate change is less reliable, shorter, and later rains. The consequence is that the window of opportunity to plough and plant is decreased, and if someone is sick at the crucial time then this can be catastrophic as no crops will be harvested for a year. Ironically, in 2006 and 2007 the rains in Malawi were good, resulting in excellent harvests.

Of course, there is an additional irony for all subsistence agriculturalists. At the beginning of the agricultural year, the farmers scan the heavens anxiously awaiting the rains that will allow them to go to their fields. But rain brings the mosquitoes and malaria and the waterborne diseases which further affect the health, especially of those with weaker immune systems.

Families and households

The first consequence of an infection is stress. No matter who is HIV positive, the question is: how did they come to be infected? Stories from across the world tell of the devastation an HIV diagnosis can bring. Because HIV is often identified through antenatal testing or when an infant is sickly, the infection is gendered – women are first to be diagnosed, and so they are assumed to have brought it into the family. At worst, it can lead to bitter family break-up. Those who argue for massive voluntary testing campaigns underestimate the stigma and shame associated with what is, after all, a deadly sexually transmitted infection.

Illness initially affects individuals. Adults who are unwell can't engage in productive work, including paid and unpaid employment as well as housework and childcare. It means people are less able to engage in community activities, the weft and warp of social reproduction. But it is not just the labour of sick adults that is lost, they in turn need care, which takes time and resources. Some help may be provided through state social and medical services, but where this is not available, care has to come from the family and community. This means that spouses care for each other, children care for their parents, and the elderly tend their children and grandchildren. Most care is provided by women, and it is generally not recognized as 'real' work. The idea that families will provide care for the sick is hardly revolutionary, it happens out of necessity all the time. AIDS, however, is costly, increasingly common, and has a bleak prognosis. This disease is causing huge trauma across households and communities.

The inability of an adult to work means less income or production. The initial response is to change resource use, so that if the family has been saving, it will stop, and expenditures are reduced. People eat fewer meals, with a lower range and quality of food. Possessions may be sold, or the family may borrow. If the household is forced to sell the assets used in production (ploughs, oxen, or a sewing machine, for example), chances of recovery are reduced.

Shocks to households are not unusual, and much has been written on this topic. People face droughts, earthquakes, floods, tsunamis, illness, and other catastrophes, and there are coping mechanisms that come into play. Unsurprisingly, the better resourced a household is at the outset, the better it will be able to cope. What makes AIDS different is that long periods of illness put a strain on even the richest. In Zambia, households with a chronically ill member have reductions in annual income of 30–35%, and where the male head of household dies, the income falls by up to 80%. Treatment is expensive, and even where drugs are provided free there are additional costs, from transport to the clinic, to ensuring the patient has an adequate diet. Thus the stark choice may be between eating and obtaining medication.

As the pandemic progresses, the burden is increasingly falling on the older women, particularly maternal grandparents. Many people in the final stages of illness return home to be cared for by parents, bringing their children. Work in Warwick Junction in Durban by May Chazan found that older women are unevenly and increasingly burdened by AIDS, bearing the brunt of the social, care-taking, economic, and emotional demands in their

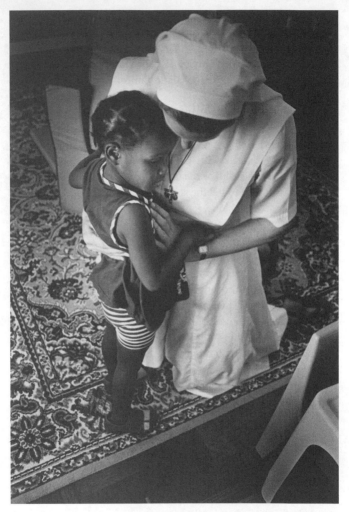

11. A nun comforting a child in an orphanage in Cape Town, South Africa, which looks after abandoned children afflicted with HIV/AIDS

families. Two-thirds of those interviewed had cared for family members or neighbours sick with AIDS. The older women in this study suffered from (largely untreated) chronic illnesses such as diabetes, arthritis, and hypertension and feared personal illness, not just for themselves, but because of what it would mean for their families. The burning question is what happens when today's grandmothers die; AIDS means the next generation of grandmothers will be absent.

In general, it is at the household level that the worst impacts of AIDS are visible. One of the main factors which exacerbates the impoverishment of people is the burden of care, providing for orphans and sick adults, which is a major expenditure and diversion of labour. Most affected households do not, in an identifiable sense, 'cope', but rather they 'struggle', and they do this because they have no other choice. In addition, households, especially rural ones, are obliged to carry the burden that is 'shifted' from the formal sector and urban areas. The unstated assumption is that 'wider society' will carry the burden: 'wider society' in this context is chiefly women in urban slums and rural areas, and they are reaching breaking point.

Development goals

Development is about more than economic growth. The UNDP's first *Human Development Report*, published in 1990, stated: 'The real wealth of a nation is its people. And the purpose of development is to create an enabling environment for people to enjoy long, healthy and creative lives.' This introduced the Human Development Index (HDI), a simple composite index constructed from three indices: life expectancy, educational attainment, and the standard of living.

The UNDP did not consider the effect of HIV/AIDS on life expectancy until 1997. When it did, the effects were dramatic – HDI scores and rankings in many countries fell significantly. Botswana dropped from 71st rank in the HDI in 1997 to 131st in 2003. Its HDI went from a peak of 0.681 in 1990 to 0.565 in 2003. By comparison, the UK's index was 0.883 in 1990 and 0.939 in 2003, and that of the USA 0.916 and 0.944 respectively. Even lower prevalence countries have been affected: Thailand fell from 52nd place in 1997 to 76th place in 2000.

In 2000 the international development targets, Millennium Development Goals (MDGs), for 2015 were set at the United Nations. These goals were to be realistic and achievable, but a 2005 progress report found movement towards these goals was not encouraging, especially for the poorest countries.

The worst affected goal is child mortality. Countries afflicted by AIDS, especially in Southern Africa, have seen increases in deaths in children under five years of age. At current rates, child mortality will be reduced by 15% by 2015, not the two-thirds target. Goal 6 is specifically to combat the three diseases of AIDS, malaria, and tuberculosis. However, they remain the primary cause of premature death in some of the poorest countries. Tuberculosis is on the rise in Africa and parts of the former Soviet Union, largely as a result of HIV/AIDS.

Although we are in the third decade of the epidemic, there is little appreciation of what HIV/AIDS means for development targets. Indicators do not pick up the impact of the disease, because they are based on historical data and take no account of current and future impact. Those who prepare the data do not compare 'with' and 'without' AIDS scenarios. Development targets and measures of 'development' need to be revised in the light of HIV/AIDS. The gendered and local nature of the epidemic must be understood.

Chapter 6
AIDS and politics

HIV/AIDS mixes sex, death, fear, and disease in ways that can be interpreted to suit different prejudices and agendas. AIDS was (and is) used to stigmatize groups. Health responses to epidemic outbreaks focus on the technical and scientific answers. The popular images are of squads of epidemiologists arriving in villages and locating the source of disease – civet cats, bats, birds – and medical task teams appearing to dispense pills and injections. We want to believe there are quick technical scientific solutions: if there are, then we can buy them, use them, and move on. This is not the case, particularly with HIV/AIDS, and rather we need to understand the underlying causes, as discussed in Chapter 3. Providing good health is not easy; it is messy and about sustainable development, equity, and justice. It needs political engagement.

AIDS is politicized. This was especially true in Southern Africa: the controversial perspectives of some senior South African political leaders, and the reasons, are explored in the text box below. The idea of AIDS as a security threat was raised in 2000 in the UN Security Council. The 'securitization' of the disease, especially in the military sense, was overstated. However, in the context of broader human security, impact is great and far-reaching.

The political implications of AIDS have received little attention. The chapter looks at how the disease is affecting representation, election processes, and political engagement, and instances of social mobilization in response to the epidemic. Finally, it looks at government, governance, and delivery at the national and international levels. AIDS is damaging the ability to deliver. Current international health governance falls short in providing leadership and direction.

The numbers game

The early history of HIV was driven by media hype. How many cases were there? Where were they? Who was being infected, and why? The first cases in the West were identified in groups of people who shared behaviours – gay men and drug users; specific nationalities – Haitians in the US; or those who received contaminated blood products – haemophiliacs and blood transfusion recipients. As the ways in which HIV is transmitted were understood, the focus shifted from identifiable categories of people to identifiable behaviours.

The epidemiology and data were introduced in Chapter 1. Initially, the data were highly political. No country wanted to be identified with the epidemic. The most blatant example of cooking the figures was in the late 1980s. Zimbabwe had officially notified the WHO that it had several hundred cases of AIDS. When South Africa first reported, it notified the WHO of 120 cases. Within days, Zimbabwe revised its figure to 119, not wanting to exceed the number reported by the racist regime to the south. Another response was simply to deny the figures. India did this by refusing to allow UNAIDS to publish an estimate of total infections in the 2004 global report. In 2006, the Ethiopian government followed suit, only allowing UNAIDS to publish a range of the estimated number of HIV infections, not the total number.

In South Africa, there has been constant debate as to how many people are actually infected. The highest figure from the Department of Health estimated there were 5.54 million infections in 2005; the lowest, from Statistics South Africa (the body charged with collecting and publishing national data), was 4.5 million; in between come the estimates from the Actuarial Society of South Africa and the Human Sciences Research Council. Does size matter? It does if data debates prevent action or provide an excuse for inaction. Once there is a generalized epidemic, more important are the number of new infections, the incidence, and consequent demand for treatment and care.

Numbers matter for funders. PEPFAR is providing US$ 15 billion, over 5 years, to 15 countries to prevent 7 million HIV infections; provide antiretroviral treatment for 2 million; and care for 10 million infected and affected people. PEPFAR's record-keeping was criticized in an April 2006 report by the US Government Accountability Office. It suggested that the programme failed to keep basic records and both under-counted and over-counted. This is important because the numbers allow Congress to track progress towards specific targets, which influences the flow of money.

The scale of the epidemic matters at the global level. In the 2006 UNAIDS report, estimates of infections were lower than those published six months previously. The decrease is ascribed to new data from the Demographic and Health Surveys and better antenatal clinic data. Will this mean that AIDS gets fewer resources, or other diseases and causes should get higher priority? Decisions as to where to put resources are dependent on more than data – they are political and economic – but numbers do matter.

HIV/AIDS, conflict, and security

The concept of HIV/AIDS as a security risk was put forward in the early 1990s. I was one of those who made this argument. We said AIDS was linked with conflict because armed forces (regular armies, militias, and rebels) had high HIV prevalence, and were more likely to engage in risky sexual behaviours and rape. Economies would be affected; development would slow down or even be reversed; and there would be substantial loss of skilled people and leadership. AIDS, therefore, had to have potential security implications.

The link between AIDS and security became a rallying cry. In 1999, the American Ambassador to the UN, Richard Holbrooke, visited Lusaka and was confronted by the issue of AIDS orphaning. This epiphany is believed to have influenced the January 2000 statement to the UN Security Council by US Vice President Al Gore. He said: 'it (HIV) threatens not just individual citizens, but the very institutions that define and defend the

Understanding South African denialism

Why did President Mbeki question the cause of AIDS? Why was the government so slow to roll out ARTs? Why did Minister of Health Tshabalala-Msimang have a fixation with nutrition, beetroot, garlic, olive oil, and lemons? These questions are posed to all South Africans engaged in HIV/AIDS work. Possible explanations include:

- The issues of sexuality and masculinity faced by all African men – including the author. AIDS threatens our construction of ourselves; having multiple partners may be seen as a 'right and reward' for being male, but it may literally cost one one's life.

- The origin of AIDS is seen by some as stigmatizing. A poor knowledge of the facts can lead to such incorrect conclusions as 'HIV comes from monkeys and HIV is sexually transmitted: therefore Africans must have had sex with monkeys'.

- HIV is sexually transmitted and African prevalence is highest. This has supported the myth that Africans can't control their sexuality. Mbeki warned of this stereotyping in the Z. K. Matthews memorial lecture at Forte Hare University in 2001.

- The politics are complex. One of history's terrible backhanders is that HIV spread as the country was liberated. Returning soldiers and exiles came from high HIV prevalence areas.

- AIDS was used by the opposition to attack government, helped by scandals: a play costing millions but achieving little; a phoney cure; the Presidential Panel to investigate the link between HIV and AIDS; and the emphasis on nutrition as opposed to medicines.

- Science and race were bound together by apartheid, which used science to its own ends; few black people had access to scientific education.

- Early messages about HIV came from the apartheid government.

- HIV/AIDS is expensive. Use of resources here meant that other expenditures could not be undertaken. Perhaps, in a Stalinist mindset, some felt AIDS was inevitable and society could become stronger for having gone through it.

- The press painted the government, President, and Minister of Health into a corner. They could do nothing right.

Yet South Africa mobilized domestic resources for HIV/AIDS. Year after year the amount of money in the budget rose. The problem lay in implementation. At the end of 2006, Vice-President Mlambo-Ngcuka took control of the AIDS programme. In mid-2007 a new National Strategic Plan, developed with wide consultation and endorsement, was released, heralding a new era.

character of a society. This disease weakens workforces and saps economic strength. AIDS strikes at teachers, and denies education to their students. It strikes at the military, and subverts the forces of order and peacekeeping.' Six months later, the Security Council passed Resolution 1308, which stated: 'the HIV/AIDS pandemic, if unchecked, may pose a risk to stability and security'.

Increased orphaning was particularly viewed as a potential threat. Children who grew up unloved, uncared for, and unsocialized were thought more likely to become criminals or even child soldiers. There are indeed many more orphans and street children, and societies and communities are stretched, but the doom-laden predictions have not materialized.

Intuitively it seemed situations of conflict would facilitate HIV spread, but limited evidence suggests the post-conflict period poses greater risk. As Pulitzer Prize-winning science writer Laurie Garrett points out, the idea that war spreads HIV does not stand up to scrutiny. In a time of conflict there may be less

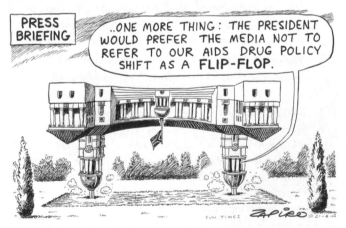

12. AIDS drug policy flip-flop

spread of communicable disease: trade decreases; borders close; and mobility, apart from refugees and armies, is diminished. It is peace, with renewed movement of people and reconstruction, that poses a bigger risk.

Recently I, with colleagues Alex de Waal and Tsadkan Gebre-Tensae, published an assessment of the risks of infection in militaries. The idea that military populations have a higher prevalence of HIV than male civilian populations does not hold at the aggregate level, although it may be true for older soldiers. Armed forces are primarily made up of young men, and male HIV prevalence rises with age. Most militaries test recruits (although few admit it), and some may test repeatedly. Being HIV positive usually excludes a person from recruitment and may result in their service being terminated. Armed forces can educate and control, and could even 'grow' an infection-free workforce.

The challenge is losing senior, experienced and skilled personnel, who are difficult to replace. Smooth functioning depends on the availability and fitness of individuals in key positions, such as the technicians who service aircraft or quartermasters. However, the military has features to minimize these impacts, including built-in redundancy: an army expects to lose individuals, usually on account of combat. A military hierarchy resembles a flattened pyramid: at every layer there are too many candidates for promotion; staff attrition is expected.

Analysts, including senior army officers, suggested, in the early years of the epidemic, that HIV/AIDS might undermine military effectiveness. The Ugandan army in the late 1980s and early 1990s under President Obote may have been affected in this way. There have been reports of some African countries having difficulty in putting together units for peacekeeping operations due to HIV in their ranks, though these are mostly anecdotal and solid evidence has still to be produced.

Most analyses of AIDS and national security appear to consist largely of a catalogue of reasons why the epidemic *may* lead to all kinds of crises. Such warnings were appropriate in the 1990s, when there were few data and much complacency. There are more data now, although they are still not being properly analysed and interpreted. This has been well documented by academics Tony Barnett and Gwyn Prins of the London School of Economics in their UNAIDS report *HIV/AIDS and Security: Fact, Fiction & Evidence*. This points to the use of 'factoids' – frequently reported statements which then are deemed to be truth – as has been the case too often with HIV/AIDS and security links.

Human security

Earlier chapters assessed the demographic impact of AIDS and showed how the disease creates poverty and despair and erodes institutional capacity. Could this epidemic cause state collapse? Disease can have this impact, as was documented for the post-Columbian Americas, when the Aztec and Inca civilizations vanished.

What happens with AIDS in the worst scenarios? In Botswana, it was predicted in 2002 that, in the absence of dramatic behaviour change or scientific advances, 80% of 15-year-old boys would die of AIDS (mortality would be even higher for girls but was not publicized as it was deemed 'too depressing'). In Swaziland, life expectancy is only 31.3 years and will decline further, infant and child mortality are rising, and the proportion of orphans will increase. In these settings, state collapse must be a real possibility.

Political scientists Andrew Price-Smith and John Daly directly implicate the epidemic in the disintegration of Zimbabwe. They argue that AIDS operates simultaneously across various domains to destabilize states and threaten their national security. Zimbabwe faces many crises: economic contraction, political corruption, failed land reform and collapse of agricultural production, environmental change, and runaway inflation. AIDS is a powerful stressor with an additional negative impact. This theme was explored for Malawi in Chapter 5. That country's plight is described as a 'perfect' storm that brings together climatic disaster, population pressure, poor governance, impoverishment, the AIDS pandemic, the long-standing burden of malaria, and other communicable diseases.

What will it take for HIV/AIDS to tip a country into collapse? What do we mean by 'collapse'? Zimbabwe continues to exist, as does Malawi. South Africa and Uganda have seen economic growth and nation-building despite the epidemic. AIDS is not seen as a cause of state failure because: the impact of the epidemic is still to be felt; societies are resilient, surprisingly so, and while we have yet to see a country disintegrate, deep and increasing poverty and misery are clearly evident; and life is messy – how do we sort the impact of AIDS from the many other stressors that these people and countries face?

The question is how many people are infected, and who are they? At certain levels of prevalence the human security impact will be limited: there are 600,000 Thais living with HIV, but in a population of 65 million that is not many, and it is hard to show that the Thai economy as a whole has been affected, though of course, the deaths of these people will affect their families, and some are devastated. A million Mozambicans or Chinese may not 'count' as a significant loss. If those falling ill and dying are not contributing to or making demands on their national economies, their passing may not be noticed by those who do 'count'. The conflict between human rights and 'real politics' and 'real economics' is only now being explored, and AIDS is one reason this is happening.

Where adult HIV prevalence is below 15%, available evidence suggests societies and economies survive economically and politically. If AIDS primarily affects the poor and the marginal, then it may not be the crisis driver predicted. But, for countries like Botswana, Swaziland, Zimbabwe, and Lesotho, survival may be moot. It is only over the next ten years that we will have a clearer idea of how countries survive or fail.

The political impact

The realization that AIDS might have political impact is comparatively recent. Political scientists were slow to engage, partly because empirical data are scarce. The data-driven thinking comes from the Democracy in Africa Research Unit (DARU) at the University of Cape Town and the South African NGO, IDASA's governance and AIDS programme. IDASA and DARU collaborate with the University of Michigan on the Afro-barometer project measuring the social, political, and economic atmosphere in Africa through national public attitude surveys. The first surveys from 1999 to 2001 were conducted in 12 countries, and by the third round there were 18 countries involved.

Political fall-out may be felt through loss of leaders and voters, changing voting patterns, and disengagement and disillusionment with the political process. Of course, all are interlinked and interact with demographics, the economy, and poverty.

In the early years, the people at greatest risk were men with money and power (and of course their partners), people who are also more likely to engage in transactional sex. Unfortunately, male political leaders fall into the category of having cash and clout, and some regard 'access' to young women as a perk of the office. There is evidence of increased mortality among politicians. In Zambia, between 1964 and 1984 there were 14 by-elections caused by deaths of parliamentarians; between 1984 and 2003 there were 59 deaths; 39 between 1993 and 2003, when AIDS mortality was increasing. By-elections are expensive, costing $200,000 in Zambia. The new representatives don't have experience and there may be less engagement between themselves and their constituents. Political parties and structures face an impact on their functioning, as loss of institutional memory and experience is pervasive.

The focus above is on national parliaments, but AIDS is felt at all tiers, including local government from province or district to municipality or town. It will also have an effect on other non-elected leaderships including chieftaincies and traditional leaders. AIDS illness and death affects those charged with planning and conducting elections. Civil servants and electoral commission officers are not immune to infection, and the nature of their work and mobility may result in greater exposure to risk.

Impact on voter numbers and engagement manifests itself in different ways. Most obvious is increased mortality. South Africa maintains a voters' roll. Analysis by IDASA shows prior to the 2004 election some 1.5 million deceased voters had been removed from the roll. The rate at which this is happening is increasing: 215,000 in 1999 rising to 358,000 in 2003, and mortality was higher among women voters. Over the same period the number of registered voters in the 18 to 19 age group fell by 49% for women and 54.7% for men. An analysis of the 2004 South African election suggested high HIV prevalence was correlated with a low turnout of young women voters.

Death is the measurable event, but illness is playing an increasing role. Sick people may not register or get to polling stations, and carers face similar problems. If people are increasingly ill or engaged in caring, levels of political engagement may decrease – citizens simply do not have the time, energy, or inclination to be involved. It is believed that participation in democracy is a 'good thing', but lower turnouts de-legitimize the process. AIDS could make a difference if it tips power balances, for instance where one ethnic or religious group has higher prevalence than another, and the voting is on ethnic or religious lines, as may occur, for example, in countries with both Muslim and non-Muslim populations such as Nigeria and some East African states.

HIV/AIDS could be important as a political or election issue, although this has not happened yet. Indeed in the Afro-barometer surveys, the primary problem identified is unemployment. In the first round of surveys, we were surprised to find HIV/AIDS featured prominently on the public agenda of only three Southern African countries: 24% of Batswana, 14% of Namibians, and 13% of South Africans cited HIV/AIDS as one of the top three problems facing their country. In contrast, just 4% of Zimbabweans, 2% of Malawians, and fewer than 1% of Basotho mentioned it as something government should address. Even more puzzling was that public prioritization of HIV/AIDS did not vary with the actual extent of the epidemic. However, 'health', including HIV, is growing in importance.

HIV/AIDS might lead to the development of broad social movements. The Treatment Action Campaign (TAC) in South Africa has been held as a model of such an organization. Many members of the TAC argue, though, that they are loyal African National Congress members and their disagreement with government is only around HIV/AIDS. In South Africa, where we would expect AIDS to be highly politicized, it has not been an election issue. In other settings AIDS has apparently been used to stigmatize candidates. For example, ahead of the March 2001 election in Uganda, *Time* magazine published an article quoting President Museveni saying of presidential candidate Dr Besigye: 'Besigye is suffering from AIDS.'

At the time of writing there are numerous examples of grassroots responses to the epidemic, from nutrition to orphan care. There are home-based care groups, and lobbying and advocacy movements pressing for reduced drug prices. However, these are still to unite politically and there are few examples of health being the driver for such mobilization.

While the direct links between AIDS and politics may be hard to identify and measure, there is cause for concern about the indirect ones. Social scientists identify three key factors for sustaining and consolidating democratic rule. First, it is harder for poor countries to maintain democracy, and contracting economies and growing inequality severely threaten democratic processes. Second, there need to be strong political institutions including civil services, judiciaries, and executives. Third are the attitudes – people must want democracy. AIDS could affect all these factors.

Government and delivery

Increased illness and death does not just affect political process. It will also influence government, particularly the civil service. Civil servants are paid less than they might be in equivalent roles in the private sector, and they expect other forms of compensation: security, sick leave, pensions, and better benefits, including death benefits. In some developing countries a civil servant can anticipate, in the event of chronic illness, six months of sick leave with full pay followed by six months on half pay. This may be further prolonged as terminating employment may require a medical board to be convened. State pensions may be paid to the wives and children of those who die in service. Under normal circumstances, these benefits should be affordable; AIDS makes the circumstances abnormal. In most workforces the mortality rate would be about 0.4%; approximately 4 in every 1,000 workers will die in a given year. Analysis of employment data suggests that AIDS increases this to between 3% and 6%, between 30 and 60 workers per 1,000.

Abnormal illness or deaths among civil servants mean government efficiency is reduced, affecting service delivery at all levels, from the schools and hospitals to the ministries. If there are no agricultural extension workers, then output in the agricultural sector will suffer as farmers lack input and advice. The illness of a customs officer may mean that goods are not cleared, an industrial process slows down, and the competitiveness of the country declines. And of course many of the best people are poached by international agencies and NGOs, paying salaries well above those of government.

Data on absenteeism and deaths in the public sector and their effects are surprisingly hard to obtain. In Malawi, absenteeism was due to personal illness, caring for sick people, and attendance at funerals. The police service saw the number of days lost due to illness increase two and half times from 1993 to 2000. The CIHD analysed personnel records for professionals in parts of the judiciary in Zambia between January 2002 and August 2005, and found that chronic disease caused annual attrition of 4.4% in the court system. Many court cases had to be adjourned because of illness, and the risk that a case would be dismissed (rather than reaching a verdict) increased by 3.5 times when illness caused adjournments.

There has been analysis of the effect of AIDS on the demand for services (increased requirements for health care, the needs of orphans, food insecurity) and the ability to provide (the change in health and education workforces, growing demands on the budget). One area that has not been researched is the effect of AIDS on revenue streams: how will AIDS affect the tax base and the ability to collect revenue?

International governance

The AIDS epidemic has given rise to a new United Nations agency (UNAIDS), and a new international funding mechanism, the Global Fund. It has resulted in bilateral aid funding flows being increased and redirected. When in January 2003, US President Bush announced PEPFAR, the US$ 15 billion budget was the largest sum ever promised to respond to a disease.

AIDS was the first disease to be debated in the Security Council and has consistently been high in global public consciousness. There are frequent meetings, and the largest, the bi-annual International AIDS Conference, attracted a record 26,000 participants in 2006. There are numerous journals and news groups serving scientists, social scientists, activists, and pressure groups. A Google search for 'AIDS information' returns 189 million hits, whereas one for 'malaria information' gets 11.3 million.

Given the intense interest and focused activity around the disease, we must ask has AIDS affected international politics and international relations? The answer is, surprisingly, not that much. The initial fears that HIV-positive people would be discriminated against, excluded from international travel, and labelled as public health menaces did not materialize. This was thanks to the activities of health and human rights activists such as the late Dr Jonathan Mann, one of the giants of the AIDS field. Mann worked as a physician and public health specialist on HIV in Kinshasa until 1986, then set up the Global Program on AIDS at WHO. In 1990 he established the François-Xavier Bagnoud Center for Health and Human Rights at Harvard University, and he was influential in the decision to switch the 1992 International AIDS Conference from Boston to Amsterdam because USA immigration authorities required HIV-positive people to declare their status. He was tragically killed in an air crash in 1998.

HIV is, correctly, not seen as a threat to the rich world, where it is generally restricted to clearly defined and mostly marginal populations. ART means those infected can be treated, so that AIDS is seen as a chronic, controllable disease. However, if growing numbers of infected people migrate into the developed countries as asylum seekers, economic migrants, or 'medical refugees' – people who can't access drugs in their own countries – this may change. In countries where access to health care is a right, there will be public debate on who receives treatment and what the rights of asylum seekers and illegal migrants are. This, and funding, will be the focus of the international politics of AIDS for the rich.

HIV/AIDS can be contrasted with SARS and avian flu. SARS effectively closed down part of Asia and Canada. A teacher from the small rural Canadian town of Perth, Ontario, described how staff were banned from travelling to Toronto at the height of the scare. Avian flu is seen as a major threat to global health and has produced similar panic. In early 2006 in Toronto, I saw packs being marketed to protect travellers against infectious disease (by implication avian flu) – each pack contained a mask, a pair of medical gloves, two antiseptic hand wipes, two antimicrobial wipes, and a thermometer!

Providing treatment for HIV/AIDS is big business. In mid-2005 there were an estimated 350,000 people on ART in Europe and these drugs have to be taken for life. The WHO estimated in mid-2006 that 6.8 million people in low- and middle-income countries would benefit from ART and 1.65 million people (24%) were getting treatment. The access to, and costs of, treatment are discussed in Chapter 7. The politics of AIDS treatment is linked with human rights, foreign assistance, and business. Providing drugs, carrying out research, and working with trade agreements and patent law are complex issues and part of international health governance.

International aid for HIV/AIDS programmes has grown substantially. An analysis of foreign aid presented by Washington-based researchers from the Center for International and Strategic Studies and the Kaiser Foundation at an international meeting in Paris in March 2006 showed that total commitments grew from US$ 63 million to US$ 104.4 million between 2000 and 2004 (however, this does not consider the fall in the value of the dollar and inflation). As a proportion of aid the funding for health increased more slowly from US$ 8.5 billion to US$ 13.5 billion.

Money gives rise to governance issues. There is a significant gap between commitments and actual spending. Indeed, when promises are tracked it becomes evident that the same pounds, dollars, or euros may be promised repeatedly by politicians. The PEPFAR commitment was unusual because so much was new (US$ 9 billion). Money comes with strings attached. These include what Americans call 'pork-barrel' issues, making sure that 'your' consultants and suppliers get the contracts – this is straightforward 'business'. But funds also flow in 'silos' for prevention or treatment, for AIDS or TB. There are issues of accounting and reporting, and each donor has their own requirements. Then there is the question of sustainability. Aid flows are partly dictated by fashion – this decade AIDS, next environmental issues?

Recently, ideology has come to the fore; programmes get preference if they promote certain issues, such as abstinence, or can't attract funding if they promote others, such as needle exchange. Originally the US Congress required that 55% of PEPFAR money should be for treatment, 15% for palliative care, 20% for HIV/AIDS prevention, and 10% for orphans and vulnerable children. Of prevention money one-third was to be spent on 'abstinence until marriage' programmes. Half the money for orphans had to be channelled through non-profit, non-governmental organizations, including faith-based organizations.

Global health governance is in a parlous state, with weak leadership and little coordination. Public health is simply not on the agenda. Responses are geared to imminent threats and not ones in the future. The WHO should be the place to look for leadership, but at the moment it is neither respected nor well run. Because it answers to the member states, it is difficult to envisage how it might change. UNAIDS offers some hope but has insufficient resources and constantly has to fight the danger of becoming bureaucratic.

Conclusion

At the moment, HIV/AIDS is the global health issue receiving the most attention and funding. At the World Economic Forum in Davos in January 2006, Nigerian President Olusegun Obasanjo, UK Chancellor Gordon Brown, and philanthropist Bill Gates called for world leaders to rally behind a major new action plan to treat 50 million people and prevent 14 million tuberculosis deaths worldwide over the next ten years. The initial cost was estimated at US$ 56 billion. In the same month, a meeting in Beijing called for US$ 1.2 billion to combat avian flu – and US$ 1.9 billion was pledged. Each disease has its advocates, and while AIDS dominates currently, this will change.

The politics of providing good health are not simple. HIV and AIDS are prime examples of where our responses have fallen miserably short of what is needed. AIDS provides a chance to examine global health governance and make changes. It is not, in the bigger picture, a threat to global security or economic development, but will become a long-term international problem that we will come to live with and accept at a global level.

At the local level, AIDS puts the continued existence of the worst affected countries in doubt. African societies where the population goes into decline, life expectancy plummets, most children are either orphaned or live in families that have taken in orphans, and where the gender balance by age changes dramatically, cannot function in a way that we consider to be 'normal'. In former Soviet countries, the high levels of infection among 'scarce' young people will have severe consequences. For families and communities, AIDS has devastating impacts.

Chapter 7
Responding to HIV/AIDS

This chapter documents responses to HIV/AIDS. It also looks at constraints: the invisibility of the epidemic; its long-wave nature; stigma; issues of sustainability and choice; and lack of resources in many affected areas.

The early reaction was mixed. Many countries took the threat seriously; in other locations complacency and denial were commonplace. Almost everywhere there were public education campaigns, and in some places attempts to target the core transmitters, particularly sex workers and IDUs.

The initial lack of medical options meant issues of public health, human rights, and development came to the fore, even if they were not framed in this way. If infected people could not be cured or treated, then how could infections be prevented? The response changed post-1996 with the development of treatments and the fall in drug prices.

There have been consistent themes over the past 25 years: scientific advances and an inability to get prevention right. The virus is intensively studied and the hunt for new drugs, vaccines, and microbicides continues. Prevention remains a challenge and the importance of gender, sexuality, and the underlying drivers of the epidemic needs attention.

The early years: limited responses

The first reaction was the scramble to identify the pathogen and how it was transmitted. The medical community, which had found itself looking on helplessly as patients died, desperately sought treatments that would work.

As soon as blood transfusions and blood products were identified as a transmission route, steps were taken to reduce this threat of infection. People at risk of HIV infection were discouraged from donating blood. In January 1985, the US Food and Drug Administration approved the first commercial HIV test. In Britain, routine blood testing began in October 1985. Ensuring safe blood was a relatively simple, technical response, and many countries rapidly put the necessary measures in place. However, in some settings, particularly where blood donors are paid (India and China are examples), HIV transmission through this route was, and remains, a major issue.

IDUs who share injecting equipment were identified early as being at risk. The approaches ranged from cracking down on drugs and users, which tended to drive people underground, to making an illegal activity safer. This latter option included campaigns to ensure users, at least, cleaned and sterilized their equipment (simple bleach worked); and at best, programmes incorporated needle exchanges, where old used needles were exchanged for new ones. The first needle exchange was introduced in February 1986 in the Scottish city of Dundee. Such successful interventions brought the IDU epidemic under control in Britain and much of Europe.

Governments saw they had a responsibility to educate and protect the broader population. The Conservative government of the UK under Prime Minister Margaret Thatcher introduced one of the earliest and most effective public information campaigns in March 1986 with the slogan 'Don't Aid AIDS'. This was followed,

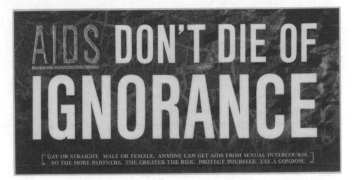

13. Anti-AIDS advertising

in January 1987, by a major advertising campaign with the catchphrase 'Don't Die of Ignorance', and a leaflet was delivered to every household in Britain. A similar campaign in Australia featured the 'Grim Reaper' in a television commercial that showed death mowing down victims in a bowling alley.

The early public education messages aimed to scare people into talking about the disease and becoming aware that they too could be at risk of infection. In the rich world much early activism was motivated by articulate and organized gay men. At a gathering in 1981, a number of homosexual men met in the New York apartment of writer Larry Kramer to discuss the 'gay cancer' and how to respond to it. This gave rise to the organization 'Gay Men's Health Crisis', followed by others such as 'ACT UP' (the AIDS Coalition To Unleash Power) and the Terrence Higgins Trust in the UK. Grassroots initiatives established in poor countries included The AIDS Support Organization (TASO) in Uganda, and the Chikankata home-based care initiative in Zambia.

In the USA, the public campaigns were mostly driven by activists and local (state and municipal) government. There was great concern in major federal health agencies such as the National

Institutes of Health and the Centers for Disease Control, but political leadership was slow to react. It was not until 1985 that President Reagan publicly mentioned HIV. Only in 1988 was there significant action when the federal government mailed 107 million copies of a booklet, *Understanding AIDS* by the Surgeon General C. Everett Koop. To his credit, Koop saw his primary function as protecting the health of Americans, not moralizing. The Bush Administration's opposition to needle exchange and emphasis on abstinence provided a troubling contrast.

Internationally, the lead was taken by the WHO's Global Programme on AIDS (GPA) under Jonathan Mann. Teams visited most developing countries, establishing Short Term Programmes on HIV/AIDS, which evolved into Medium Term Programmes run by national AIDS control offices. The emphasis was on risk reduction through information and education. People were encouraged to understand and change their behaviours. Condoms were distributed, testing and counselling made available, and occasionally, where appropriate, needle exchange programmes set up.

It was recognized that programmes needed to look beyond individual risks and understand that behaviours take place in a social, political, and economic environment (see Chapter 3). In every society, regardless of where and how the epidemic enters, those who are marginalized, stigmatized, and discriminated against are at greatest risk. Sadly, the WHO failed to sustain the leadership and imagination needed to tackle the epidemic. The response – outside the GPA – was technical, treating the epidemic as primarily a health problem. It was hampered by the distaste for the sexual nature of the disease. All international agencies, from the Food and Agriculture Organization (FAO) to the World Bank, consistently underestimated the potential scale of the epidemic.

In building the GPA, Mann bypassed many entrenched interests, bringing him into conflict particularly with Dr H. Nakajima,

WHO Director-General from 1988. In 1990, Mann resigned in protest over the way he and the issue of HIV/AIDS were being sidelined. However, the importance of AIDS led, in the early 1990s, to the establishment of UNAIDS, as a joint programme, initially of WHO, UNICEF, UNDP, UNESCO, UNFPA, and the World Bank. This began operating, under the leadership of Dr Peter Piot, in January 1996.

It is noteworthy that the most effective early responses to the epidemic were 'home-grown'. In Thailand, HIV prevention and control became a top priority in 1991/2, under the unelected government of Prime Minister Anand Panyarachun. The wake-up call was concern that the epidemic might have major economic impacts, especially on tourism. An AIDS policy was put in place under the Office of the Prime Minister with a multi-sectoral National AIDS Prevention and Control Committee chaired by the Prime Minister. A massive public information campaign began, and the '100% condom programme' required mandatory condom use in all commercial sex establishments. Prostitutes were screened at government sexually transmitted disease clinics and issued with free condoms. Male patients were asked who they had had sex with. If they were infected in a brothel, it was assumed to be non-compliant, and could be closed.

In Senegal, following the first AIDS case in 1986, a National AIDS Programme was established with strong political support. Religious leaders played a crucial role, with Islamic organizations becoming involved as early as 1989 and imams giving public support to AIDS-prevention activities. Commercial sex work was legal and licensed so could be regulated.

Most controversial was prevention in Cuba. In the 1980s, the authorities tested the entire population, isolating those found to be HIV positive in 'sanatoria'. They continued testing returning migrants. At the end of 2005, there were only about 4,200 infected Cubans. This draconian approach required a high degree of governmental control, a compliant population, and non-porous borders, and was never an option for most countries. It was tried in the former Soviet Union, with massive campaigns of testing for everyone who could possibly have been exposed to the virus. Apart from the expense and difficulty of implementing such a programme, many argue it violates human rights. The 'opt-out' testing in Botswana and door-to-door testing in Lesotho, discussed later, are an uneasy compromise.

In the examples above, HIV spread was successfully prevented. Uganda was the first country to bring prevalence down. At its peak, in the late 1980s, prevalence there was 35% in some groups, and currently among adults it is estimated at 6.7%. The reasons have been extensively debated. The religious right argues it is due to behaviour change, social marketers advise condoms were critical, and others suggest it was simply the natural progression of an epidemic. What is agreed is that, for intervention to work, the early, realistic recognition of the disease was crucial. President Museveni responded proactively, fostering a multi-sectoral response. Ordinary Ugandans saw the evidence of the epidemic and responded to the messages. Non-regular partnering decreased, sexual debut was delayed, and condom use increased. Crucially, this national response worked effectively at local levels.

The shift to treatment

The emphasis from the beginning of the epidemic until 1996 was on prevention and care of the sick. There was little focus on treatment, despite the growing numbers of deaths of young adults, parents, farmers, and breadwinners. In 1996, there were major changes. In Geneva, UNAIDS began functioning. There was the announcement of new drugs at the XIth International Conference. It was hoped the drugs could completely eliminate the virus from a patient's body, and while this optimism proved unfounded, treatment can turn AIDS into a chronic, manageable disorder.

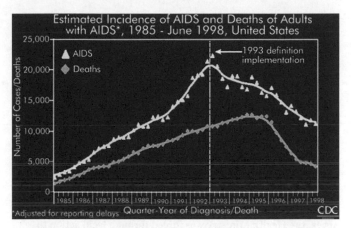

14. Adult mortality trends in the USA

Initially, costs of treatment were phenomenal – a minimum of US$ 12,000 per patient per year. Treatment was not easy: there were unpleasant side effects; patients had to take large numbers of tablets, some with food and some on an empty stomach; and some drugs had to be kept in cold storage. For most infected people, expensive drugs were far beyond their reach, but in the rich world the number of people dying fell dramatically, as shown in Figure 14.

By the end of the 1990s, with South Africa reporting the largest number of HIV infections in the world, the XIIIth International AIDS Conference was held in Durban – the first in a developing country. Nelson Mandela closed the conference with a call for action – that drugs should be made available and accessible to all.

Funding and treatment

Since 2000, the response has been dominated by new initiatives and treatments. The price of drugs fell dramatically (Figure 15). Indian companies led the way, manufacturing generic drugs at a fraction of the cost of brand names. One, Cipla, offered to

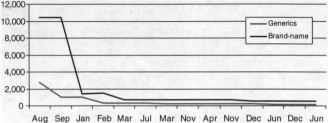

15. World prices per patient per year for simple antiretroviral treatment (US dollars)

make AIDS drugs available at less than US$ 1 per day. In South Africa, the Health Ministry was forced through legal action to supply treatment to prevent mother-to-child transmission. WHO published guidelines for providing antiretrovirals in resource-poor countries, and listed 12 essential AIDS drugs.

In 2001, the United Nation's Secretary-General, Kofi Annan, called for spending on AIDS to be increased tenfold in developing countries, and the Global Fund was established. The second major initiative was the US PEPFAR funding. The new WHO Director-General, Lee Jong-Wook, named HIV/AIDS as his top priority in his first speech, declaring the failure to deliver treatment was a global public health emergency. On World AIDS Day 2003, he announced (with UNAIDS) a new plan called '3 by 5', aiming to treat 3 million people in poor countries by the end of 2005. This target was not achieved: although the number of people on treatment tripled, it only reached 1.3 million in December 2005. At the end of 2006, an estimated 2,015,000 people in low- and middle-income countries were on ART.

Financial resources are greater than ever. In 1996, about US$ 300 million was available in low- and middle-income countries. By 2006, there was US$ 8.3 billion accessible, although this fell short of the estimated requirement of US$ 14.9 billion. UNAIDS expects, on current trends, there may be US$ 10 billion in 2007. In 2008, some US$ 22.1 billion will be needed, though there are at the time of writing no estimates of how much money will be available beyond 2008. The funding does not consider capacity, or whether or not the money will be spent effectively. The emphasis has swung towards a 're-medicalization' and technical interventions. The reasons for this are deep-seated. Availability of treatment, the decline in drug prices, and increased resources mean there is an option for medical responses. But the changing emphasis is also driven by an unwillingness to engage with the drivers of the epidemic: the social justice issues.

Despite rapid scientific advances, there are still no simple solutions. There will almost certainly not be a vaccine available by 2015, the date the Millennium Development Goals were to be met. In 2007, there were just four pharmaceutical companies with vaccines in trials; only one candidate has gone though all the processes and it was not effective. The International AIDS Vaccine Initiative points out that global spending on an AIDS vaccine is less than 1% of spending on all health product research and development.

Microbicides could prevent the sexual transmission of HIV and other STIs when applied topically. There are about 60 substances

Alternative paradigms for testing

One crucial element of intervention is for people to know their HIV status. If a person knows they are negative, they have incentives to remain so. If they test positive, they can make lifestyle changes, access services, and avoid re-infection with HIV. Uptake of voluntary counselling and testing has been slow. Two innovative approaches are being tried in Southern Africa.

In Botswana, a national programme for ART was introduced in 2003. This programme, a partnership between government, the Gates Foundation, and Merck, a drug company, found that, after an initial rush, patients were slow to come forward. Government introduced 'routine testing'. Every person attending a public health facility will be tested unless they opt out, or specifically decline. The evidence is that close to 90% are tested.

In Lesotho, a 'Know Your Status' campaign was launched in mid-2006. Teams go from door to door offering 'on the spot' testing. Those tested should be able to access counselling and support, and drugs when necessary. This programme is controversial. Early reports were that some of those charged with carrying out the testing did not know their own HIV status and would be unwilling to undergo testing. There are also concerns about the ability to access follow-up services and confidentiality.

If the stigma and discrimination surrounding HIV are to be addressed, knowledge of one's HIV status and a normalization of the epidemic are essential. However, there are many issues surrounding testing, and simple 'know your status' campaigns are not sufficient. Neither is it enough to know one's HIV status. An infected person should also know their CD4 cell count, which indicates whether they need treatment, and provides a baseline for monitoring health.

being tested, but no safe and effective product is yet available. If the current research is successful, it is hoped a microbicide could be available by around 2012. Use of microbicides could be female-controlled, which is important for those for whom condoms, mutual monogamy, and STI treatment are not feasible.

The research into drugs is ongoing, and both new drugs and new combinations are being made, developed, licensed, and marketed. In June 2006, the first 'once-a-day' tablet, a combination of three drugs, was announced, making it easier for patients to comply and helping to prevent drug resistance.

In the developing world particularly, 'alternative' therapies are popular, and many people in low- and middle-income countries see traditional healers as their first line of treatment. Treatments range from nutritional supplements and immune system boosters that have been subject to scientifically rigorous research, to downright quackery with charlatans marketing potions revealed to them in dreams. Unfortunately, these therapies are not tested or licensed in the same way as conventional drugs. There is a role for alternative therapies and therapists if they are proven to help and are monitored and licensed. The challenge is for allopathic and alternative medicine to work together.

Are responses appropriate and adequate?

The responses will depend on the country and size and stage of the epidemic. The primary object must be to prevent people from being infected. Prevention has been broadly successful in rich countries, although vigilance is necessary to ensure that the epidemic does not take off in any particular groups or sub-groups. It is alarming to learn that there have been significant numbers of new HIV infections in the gay population in San Francisco. In Britain, numbers of sexually transmitted infections have been rising since the 1990s – in 2005, there were nearly 800,000 new diagnoses, a 3% increase on 2004. Worryingly, according to a National AIDS Trust survey released in 2006, people interviewed at that time were more ignorant of how HIV is spread than those surveyed in 2000. Prevention campaigns must be maintained, as new cohorts of people becoming sexually active have to be reached and educated. HIV prevention is not something that can be 'done' and ticked off a list.

Table 5. Locating appropriate responses

Type of epidemic	Stage of epidemic	Prospects for increased infections	Country examples	Response
Limited to specific groups	Early	Limited	Tunisia, Morocco	Epidemiologic vigilance
Limited to specific groups	Early	Likely	Ukraine, Indonesia	Intense targeted interventions
Limited to specific groups	Late	Limited	UK, Australia, Philippines	Continued monitoring, targeted prevention, treatment where appropriate

Spreading to general populations	Early	Limited	Senegal, Thailand	Epidemiologic vigilance, intense targeted interventions
Spreading to general populations	Early	Likely	Papua New Guinea	Intense broad interventions, care and impact mitigation
Widespread	Early	Likely	South Africa	Focus on youth, gender, care and impact mitigation
Widespread	Late	Limited	Zambia	Establish what worked and intensify activities, care, and impact mitigation

If prevention does not work, then countries must deal with the consequences. Table 5 sets out stages and types of response – this relates to the curves described in Chapter 1. Put simply, if prevention fails, more people need treatment, fall ill, and die, and these consequences must be tackled. Treatment and impact mitigation become necessary. Even in the worst affected countries, prevention must be a priority. Prevention is not working and providing treatment for increasing numbers has been described as 'mopping the floor while the tap is running'; it is neither sustainable nor affordable.

Constraints to response

Responses have been and continue to be constrained. The most fundamental problem has been getting people (especially decision-makers) to understand the nature of the epidemic and what it might do to society. In the early years, one prevention poster took as its theme an iceberg – AIDS cases represented the tip with the mass of HIV infections hidden. This illustrates the dilemma of getting people to take AIDS seriously. Given the iceberg is hidden, how can we persuade people of its presence? Unfortunately, for those who want an excuse to ignore HIV/AIDS, there are scientists and pseudo-scientists willing to provide 'evidence'.

Key questions are: how do we convince people of the existence of the epidemic where it is not yet visible; how do we deal with the stigma related to the sexual nature of HIV; what do we do about it in resource-poor settings; and how do we get a sustained global response? Where it is not yet visible, the challenge is to convince people of the danger that the epidemic poses. This means that they have to believe in the existence of the disease; understand it has the potential to spread; and will pose a credible threat. Achieving this is not easy. These issues are faced by all social and public health and safety campaigns – anti-smoking, drink driving, and seat belt campaigns provide instructive examples. They show it is possible to change behaviours, but it takes time and needs appropriate rewards and penalties.

There are helpful parallels from another global issue – climate change. Most people believe weather patterns are changing: floods, heat waves, and droughts seem increasingly common and severe. Many suspect that human activity contributes to global warming and want something to be done. Climate change is generally acknowledged and 'owned', but individuals don't know what to do. The parallels extend further: global climate change and HIV/AIDS have been recognized for about 25 years; there is a desire to find technical solutions; and not all will be affected or able to respond equally – the Maldives and Bangladesh face different problems from New Zealand or Japan. But there is also one important difference: much of the work on climate change impact is forward-looking, in the HIV/AIDS field we look back.

Most national and international leaders believe HIV exists. Unfortunately, the step from recognizing the existence of the virus to understanding how it operates and what impact it will have is not simple. Appropriate equitable responses also mean questioning what is otherwise taken for granted: why should we have to make a choice of who gets treatment? Why should wealthy Europeans get all the laboratory investigation they need to tailor their treatment, while the WHO guidelines for resource-poor settings provide an algorithm for treatment without even an HIV test?

Sex, gender, and stigma

HIV is not a contagious disease. It is not contracted by sitting next to a carrier on public transport, as might be the case with influenza, or by eating salad contaminated with bacteria, as with cholera. The cause can be identified. A person with HIV has either done something to cause the infection: had sex with an infected person, used a contaminated needle, or had a needle-stick injury.

Or they have had something done to them: been raped, born to an infected mother, or received infected blood. This leads to concepts of innocence and guilt. Stigma and blame is further compounded because many of the behaviours that lead to HIV transmission are circumscribed by society.

For people to accept HIV has the potential to spread, they must acknowledge the behaviours that allow its spread – drug use, homosexuality, men visiting commercial sex workers, sex outside of marriage, and so on. Admitting people behave in ways that allow the spread of HIV creates moral dilemmas and political problems. In all societies, injecting drug use is an illegal and socially unacceptable behaviour. In some settings, simply having more than one partner and having sex outside marriage are seen as shameful and stigmatizing, especially for women. Crucial here are gender dynamics and politics: women are often first to be identified as HIV infected; where the epidemic is heterosexually driven, more women than men are infected; and women may transmit HIV to their children.

Data show women are less likely than men to have sex with a non-marital, non-cohabiting partner. UNAIDS reported in Malawi in 2000 that over 70% of young men had sex with non-regular partners, but for women this was fewer than 20%. In Thailand in 1999, three-quarters of infected women reported sex with their husbands as their only HIV risk factor, and nearly half thought they were at no or low risk. A joint report by UNAIDS, UNFPA, and UNIFEM details how in Kisumu, Kenya, 22% of unmarried girls were HIV positive compared to 33% of married girls. In India, the primary risk factor for a woman is to be married.

For many women, the messages of 'abstain, be faithful, and use a condom' may be meaningless. Where they are forced or pressured into sexual activity, the idea of abstinence is impossible. If their partners have extra-marital sex or are infected at marriage then being faithful offers no protection. Using a condom requires contraceptive availability, and their use is controlled by men. Using condoms also may imply a lack of trust and some believe makes sex less fun. Obviously, when a couple wants to start a family, condom use has to be discontinued.

While homosexuality is accepted in some countries, in most it is stigmatized, and in several actually illegal. Homophobia at the highest level is a reality, particularly in Africa and the Caribbean. Robert Mugabe described gays and lesbians as 'worse than pigs and dogs' at a book fair in Harare in 1993. These views find resonance elsewhere. In 2001, President Sam Nujoma said: 'The Republic of Namibia does not allow homosexuality, lesbianism here. Police are ordered to arrest you, and deport you, and imprison you, too.' In Nigeria in 2006, the Federal Government banned homosexuality and lesbianism and outlawed same-sex marriage.

Infection through sex implies, among unmarried people, that they have had sex before marriage. Where people are in committed relationships, this either means one partner brought the infection into the relationship or they had sex outside of it. The moral responses that get the most 'air time' are primarily driven by the Christian Right. Issues of sexuality, especially men having sex with men, and drug use find resonance with conservatives in Africa, Eastern Europe, and Asia. The message is: 'if we follow God's teachings and don't have sex outside a single stable union, engage in gay sex or use drugs, then we are not at risk of infection'.

Humankind is constrained by a set of attitudes to sex that is unique to our species. As Jared Diamond notes in a readable little book, *Why is Sex Fun?*: 'The subject of sex preoccupies us. It's the source of our most intense pleasures. Often it is the cause of misery, much of which arrives from the built-in conflicts between the evolved roles of women and men.' Sexuality in humans has universal features that hinder our response to HIV/AIDS, and may stem from our particular biological, economic, and social evolution.

The perception that stable family units are the best way to bring up children is deeply ingrained and even institutionalized. Social norms say that people should have stable relationships with one lifetime partner and should stick to that partner sexually. People enter long-term male–female relationships with mutual obligations – the primary one is parental care of children. Humans are an exceptional species in the time we take to rear our young – young people may not vote until they are 18, and in America people must be over 21 before they are legally allowed to drink alcohol.

Couples (and this can be extended to polygamous families) live in societies made up mainly of other couples with whom they share common territory and cooperate socially and economically. Sexual experiences prior to marriage are acknowledged though not condoned. It is not generally accepted for people to have partners outside their long-term child-rearing relationship.

One of the ways we bond for the biological and social imperative of child-rearing is through sex. This is why most sexual activity is for fun not, directly, for reproduction. In these relationships, couples have sex repeatedly and mainly exclusively with each other; in private (public sex is generally a criminal offence); and not just when women are fertile. Humans evolved concealed ovulation and constant receptivity to make this combination of pairing and co-parenting possible.

There is an evolutionary paradox, though: biologically, any being's goal is to pass on their genes and that means fertilizing or being fertilized by the most desirable partner. Among some creatures, the male's contribution is simply the sperm; in others, pairing is for the season; among a few, the union is for life. In some species, males seek exclusivity over their mates, examples being herds of impala, with one male and up to 20 females, or a pride of lions. Even when pairing is apparently exclusive, infidelity occurs. If a male or female can have sex and fertilize or be fertilized by a more (in evolutionary terms) desirable partner, and not be found out (thus jeopardizing the pairing that raises the next generation), then the instinct is to do this. In human society, being caught having extra-marital sex is usually catastrophic, with potential to cause marital disruption and consequent adverse effects on parental cooperation in child rearing.

Herein is a paradox with regard to HIV and AIDS. A person who is HIV positive has almost certainly had sex with someone who is infected. Among unmarried people, this reveals sex before marriage. Where people are in relationships, an infection 'finds you out', has social consequences, and brings huge stress. It is the stigma of the epidemic, and of course it is gendered. Men try to control female reproduction, and most societies have double standards when it comes to sexuality; it is more acceptable for men to have sex before marriage, to have multiple partners, use sex workers, and have affairs.

Resource-poor settings: priorities and sustainability

In Toronto in August 2006, there was evidence of new discourses. There were two interlinked themes concerning medicine and money. The medical response is about getting people on treatment and is linked to the right to treatment. Monetary issues came to the fore in parallel with drug development, as money is needed to buy drugs and to provide staff and infrastructure to deliver them. There was also a growing realization that prevention must be higher on the agenda.

There are issues around setting priorities and ensuring the response is sustainable. Priority-setting is something we are all familiar with in our daily lives, dealing with the scarce resources of time and money. If the family budget is spent on a new car, then the summer holiday will be sacrificed; if the evening is spent playing monopoly, then the homework won't get done. Governments too make choices – if Britain spends £20 billion on a new trident nuclear submarine programme, this money is not then available for the National Health Service. We need to decide what level of resources, financial and human, should be devoted to HIV/AIDS.

Currently, considerable sums of money are pledged. However, pledges are not the same as money flows. And even when the commitments are real, spending at the country level may not happen. A looming problem is sustainability. More money may be crucial, but we are not even certain the same level of resources will be maintained into the future.

Chapter 8
The next 25 years

This concluding chapter focuses on major issues around HIV and
AIDS, including some of the uncomfortable 'realpolitik' we must
face. I believe the epidemic will receive less attention as other
concerns hit the global agenda. These include climate change;
access to energy and water resources; shifting power balances;
and new diseases.

What have we learned?

The HIV/AIDS epidemic is causing a complex systemic change
in human ecology. It is unleashing secondary impacts that
have demographic and epidemiological consequences, which in
turn create feedback loops into the dynamics of the epidemic
itself.

This Very Short Introduction argues that AIDS is a unique disease
with dreadful impacts on those places worst affected. It calls into
question whether some nations will survive its ravages. In many
African countries, the burden of care is being borne by the elderly,
but HIV means there won't be enough old people in a generation.
There are changing demographics: falling life expectancy; shifting
population structures; gender ratios altering; and growing
numbers of orphans. Some societies will change significantly,

and while this is a slow and incremental process, AIDS will be at its core.

The way the disease has spread shows the fractures and inequalities of our society; it also shows how interconnected we are. HIV emerged in Africa and spread across the globe in less than ten years. A resistant variety that materializes in New York can be transmitted in Bangkok in a matter of weeks. AIDS also shows our gains: science has made huge advances, and debates around human rights and equity have been driven by the disease.

AIDS is not a threat to the human species. It is located among the poorest and most marginalized in our society, whether they be the indigenous people of Canada; the drug users in Dublin; or entire nations, the Malawians or Swazi. This means global responses, however grounded in common sense and self-interest, need to be driven by responsibility and compassion.

AIDS is exceptional

Should AIDS be treated differently from other diseases? Should it be dealt with as a crisis or as a long-term development issue? This is an ongoing debate with no single or simple answer. Let me sum up the points I have made in this book.

AIDS is primarily a sexually transmitted infection affecting young adults. The spread is silent and the long incubation period means the virus has infected many people before illnesses manifest and the threat is apparent. Eminent British scientist Professor Roy Anderson modelled the course of the epidemic and estimated it will take 130 years to work through the global population.

There is no cure. There are treatments, but these remain relatively expensive. In poor countries, the cost of treating one AIDS patient is many times the average expenditure on health. Even if money were no object, there are human resource constraints to providing treatment. Science has made huge strides, but there will be no vaccine or microbicide available in the medium term. ↪ Author's opinion

AIDS is already having a devastating impact on some countries. In Swaziland, the chance of a 15-year-old boy living to 50 years is 28%, for a girl it is just 22%. Before AIDS, it was 92% and 97% respectively. The UNDP estimated 2004 life expectancy in Botswana to be 34.9 years. Populations in some African countries are projected to decline. Reversing life expectancies and falling populations are events unknown in the past 200 years. Economists question whether economic growth is possible in these circumstances; sociologists and political scientists have not begun to consider the ramifications.

The debate between normalization and exceptionalism is sterile. AIDS is exceptional and needs to be treated as such. But the measures needed to deal with the schisms and fractures that give rise to the epidemic are long term. Preventing AIDS means equitable development· providing education, health, employment opportunities, and social support. These are development goals, and not (just) about HIV/AIDS.

Perceptions

The innovative responses needed mean we must change perceptions. In spatial terms, the worst of the epidemic and hence its worst impacts are geographically bounded. Early fears that HIV would spread widely and uniformly were unfounded, and not all parts of the world are equally affected. Through a mixture of circumstance and predisposition, areas of Africa are particularly badly hit, though the smaller epidemics of Eastern Europe may have devastating consequences because of their demographic circumstances.

In temporal terms, AIDS shows how limited our time horizon is. Humanity has difficulty in taking long-term views. Most planning is geared to three to five year strategies. We want immediate solutions and to believe things will get better. Companies do not project declining profits; politicians do not warn of bleak futures. Humans see things in the short term and through rose-tinted glasses. But AIDS requires a long-term, realistic view. We know the number of illnesses and deaths will increase, in fact there is an awful predictability about HIV/AIDS and what it has the potential to do, and we need to get to grips with this.

Perhaps a key is to change our perspective. How would our great grandchildren see the epidemic if they were looking back from 2108? For them, HIV/AIDS will have been an historical event. If we develop this thinking, then history could provide ideas, paradigms, and methodologies for understanding and responding. There are lessons from the past we can apply; we need to learn from history and historians.

Prevention imperatives

Most important is avoiding future infections. AIDS is devastating for households, families, and society at large. Preventing infections means, in economic language, future costs will not have to be borne, additional human suffering will be averted. Prevention must remain the priority. If we knew what worked, it would be clear where resources should go, but as the book shows there are no easy answers. The drivers of the epidemic are multifaceted and responses need to take cognizance of the complexity of society, economies, and political management. We need to better understand sexuality.

There are effective targeted and technical interventions for early epidemics. This was seen in prevention of transmission through infected blood, responses to infection among drug users in Europe, and the timely interventions among sex workers in Thailand and Senegal. When the epidemic spreads beyond these populations, prevention becomes more haphazard and less successful.

There are three main lessons from the last 25 years. The first is that leadership is crucial. With strong, supportive leadership, prevention becomes possible; without it, it is extremely difficult. An editorial in *The Lancet* ahead of the 2004 International AIDS Conference in Bangkok identified the willingness of political leaders to acknowledge the crisis and implement interventions swiftly as the most important factor in changing the course of the epidemic. Uganda, Thailand, and Cambodia were singled out as countries where this happened.

The second area is gender and gender equity. Globally, HIV disproportionately infects and affects women. Not only are they more likely to be HIV positive, but they bear the burden of care and support. Prevention must empower women; give them choice over whom they have sex with, when, and how. Men must accept this and not feel threatened.

The final concerns around prevention messages are what they are and who is targeted. A narrow focus on abstinence and fidelity is unrealistic, hypocritical, and stigmatizing. The emphasis should be on responsible sexual behaviour rather than scare tactics. The discourse needs to move from sex to relationships, teaching people how to negotiate and develop responsible and loving interactions. Young people need to be inculcated with the behaviours and values that allow them to protect themselves from HIV and lead fulfilling lives. There is little point in targeting people whose sexual behaviours are set and unlikely to change. Single-component interventions do not work anywhere, and no general approach will work everywhere.

The treatment debate

When prevention fails, treatment is necessary. It is to the credit of science and activists that this is widely available and increasingly affordable. It took mobilization, militant campaigning, and legal action to bring the price of treatment within the means of poorer countries.

Treatment is still not universally accessible, nor will it be. With the current drugs and modes of administering them, there are simply not the human resources and infrastructure to provide treatment to all. For example, in 2004 Mozambique had under 800 doctors, a third of whom were foreign, fewer than 0.3 per 1,000 people. Providing ART to all who need it would need at least an additional 200 doctors plus nurses, pharmacists, and other staff. Health systems are under pressure, and staff are being diverted to AIDS.

Three key aspects of treatment are cost, sustainability, and access. The cheapest ART available is about US$ 150 per patient per year for the drugs alone. The associated testing, medical staff, and so on push the minimum cost to between US$ 200 and US$ 300. Put starkly, it costs between 0.54c and 0.82c a day to keep an infected person alive. One billion people, 19% of the world's population, live on less than a dollar a day, many in the countries worst affected by AIDS, such as Zambia, where 63% of people live on less than a dollar per day. Per capita government health expenditure, assessed in the 2006 World Health Report was US$ 3 in Nepal, US$ 6 in Nigeria, US$ 25 in Lesotho, and US$ 40 in Ukraine (in the UK, it is US$ 2,081 and the USA, US$ 2,548). In high-prevalence countries, the cost of therapy is many times the annual health budget. But it has also become apparent how complex providing ART is. There are reports of drugs being held back at ports because of unpaid duties, dispensaries running out of medicine, and people having to bribe their way into programmes.

Even with the limited treatment, there are questions of sustainability. Most treatment in the poor world is funded by donors, in particular the Global Fund and PEPFAR. At the end of March 2006, PEPFAR was supporting treatment for 561,000 men, women, and children. But PEPFAR was a five-year programme ending in 2008 with possible renewal to 2013, and the Global Fund projects too have a limited lifespan. The current challenge is to get people on treatment, but soon it will be to ensure there are the resources to continue, because patients need treatment for life.

Access is a complex issue, and choices have to be made. If not everyone can be treated, who do we treat? This debate creates huge difficulties among people working in the field of AIDS, human rights activists, and lawyers. Given that rationing is occurring, we need to ask on what basis should these decisions be made? In a seminal 2005 article in *PLoS Medicine* on rationing and its causes and consequences, Sydney Rosen and colleagues point out: 'As used by economists, rationing is a morally neutral concept. It does not imply an intent to deprive some people of a good, but rather describes the allocation of a resource of which there is not enough to go around.'

Should decisions be made on economic grounds, treating those who make the largest contribution to society first? There is a strong argument for giving health care workers preferential access – after all, they have to treat others. A WHO slogan is 'test, treat and retain'. Should treatment be made available on the basis of equity or gender? Or on the basis of some other criterion of what society wants and how it values people? There are no easy answers. Currently, decisions are made through a combination of medical imperatives, treating the sickest first; access, who can get to the treatment sites; and where the money is. Those with higher CD4 counts need the least clinical management. Using limited resources to manage crises is not optimal.

As the '3 by 5' initiative rolled out, it became apparent that providing treatment is not enough. The WHO recommended making antiretrovirals affordable and providing them free to the poor. What affordability means and who is poor are not defined. Our analysis shows that in low-income countries treatment should be free. Trying to implement user fees is a waste of scarce resources as they are costly to put in place and administer, and exemptions or waivers rarely reach those who need them. Asking the poor to pay for health care is not just impractical, it is also obscene. We looked at AIDS exceptionalism – should AIDS be treated free when other diseases are not? Other diseases are treated free where there is a public health reason to do so. Given the nature of the AIDS epidemic, providing free treatment should be an imperative even though the principle cannot be applied to all diseases or all in need.

Treatment issues also raise the question of targets. Should targets continue to be set given they won't be reached? Having a goal may be good from the perspective of a Western capitalist or activist, but some in the developing world view target-setting as a hypocritical activity because they are seldom met. This debate is broader than HIV/AIDS, it extends to the Millennium Development Goals, G8 commitments, and beyond.

Locating and dealing with impact

Much writing has described how people 'cope', but what is coping? For many it is simply struggling with increased impoverishment and misery. A household that does not access health care or child support but somehow continues to bring up its children can be said to be coping. But is this what society wants and will accept? Coping needs to be more than surviving.

The major impact is on human capital, which is increasingly recognized as critical for long-term development. It is being steadily and insidiously eroded. The illness and deaths of adults has effects across society. In government work gets done inefficiently, more slowly, or not at all. For the private sector, productivity is reduced and costs increased. Among farmers, it means there is less labour at critical times. The impact is intergenerational, as children with sick parents will not get the emotional and financial investment they need. Having a generation of orphans growing up uncared for and under-educated creates long-term problems. The long-wave complex impacts of HIV/AIDS are not appreciated.

Impact is gendered. Young women are afraid of dying and leaving their children, and they feel powerless to prevent infection. Older women, who bear the brunt of the social, care-taking, economic, and emotional burdens of the epidemic in their families, are supporting growing numbers on shrinking incomes.

Social transfers, sustainability, and the role of governments

In early 2006 at a Global Partners Forum on Children Affected by HIV and AIDS, British Deputy Minister for International Development, Gareth Thomas, identified social welfare as a core issue for debate. This means ensuring a minimum standard of living and access to essential services for all. The experience of rich countries has proven that social welfare is central to proper support for the most vulnerable, indeed free schooling and health facilities provide the basis for development. It is hypocritical to apply a different standard to poorer countries. Rather, we need to ensure social transfers, such as child benefits and social pensions, are the norm in all developing countries.

Dealing realistically with HIV prevention and AIDS does not lie only in responding to the disease but in addressing the underlying causes: poverty and inequality. This requires global reform in trade and international commitments. In the short term, social welfare programmes will go a long way to meeting the needs. But these interventions are not 'sustainable' as the word is currently used. Countries and communities won't graduate from needing support in the short or medium term, and questions of what 'sustainable development' actually is need to be posed.

Final thoughts

Adam Smith argued centuries ago that governments should provide stability and law. In fact, we can and should demand far more of our governments at both the national and international levels. There are basic rights to health, education, incomes, and shelter. If these were met, we would not have the epidemic we currently face.

It bodes ill for humankind that we do not respond adequately to HIV/AIDS. We will face many other challenges. These include new, more easily spread diseases needing innovative, rapid public health responses. We confront global equity issues such as access to water. Climate change desperately requires international and coordinated action. AIDS is a harbinger, the first of many new and alarming challenges, and has given us the opportunity to learn. Only time will tell if we did.

References and further reading

AIDS is the most studied disease in human history. The literature is huge, ranging from dense scientific writing to popular texts. In addition to published documents there are theses, press clippings, and the internet. Over the past 20 years I have read widely, hopefully reflected in the rich diversity of information and ideas I have presented. In keeping with the Very Short Introduction style I have kept quotations to a minimum. The bibliography below represents a small part of what is available and the most accessible sources.

General literature and data

The World Wide Web provides the best source of up-to-date information. The prime website is: UNAIDS www.unaids.org (where the Global AIDS Epidemic reports can be accessed). International data come from the World Health Organization www.who.org, UNDP www.undp.org, and UNICEF www.unicef.org.

Much information focusing on HIV/AIDS data and history comes from www.avert.org, an AIDS charity, and the US Centers for Disease Control www.cdc.gov. My work and that of my division can be accessed at www.heard.org.za.

My co-authored book, Tony Barnett and Alan Whiteside, *AIDS in the Twenty-First Century: Disease and Globalization*, 2nd edn (Palgrave,

2006) reviews literature on epidemiology and impact. Additional useful general texts are Gerald J. Stine, *AIDS Update 2005: An Annual Overview of Acquired Immune Deficiency Syndrome* (Pearson Benjamin Cummings, 2005); Jonathan Mann and Daniel Tarantola (eds), *AIDS in the World II* (Oxford University Press, 1996); and Salim Karim and Quarraisha Karim (eds) *HIV/AIDS in South Africa* (Cambridge University Press, 2005).

Without doubt the most sobering reflection on what pandemic disease can do to a society is Charles C. Mann, *Ancient Americans: Rewriting the History of the New World* (Granta Books, 2005). Thought-provoking books are Alex De Waal, *AIDS and Power: Why There Is No Political Crisis – Yet* (Zed Books, 2006) and Stephen Lewis, *Race against Time* (House of Anansi Press, 2005).

Chapter 1

Excellent historical accounts of the disease include Randy Shilts, *And the Band Played On: Politics, People and the AIDS Epidemic* (St Martin's Press, 1987), which describes the early years of the pandemic. An account of the African epidemic is Edward Hooper Slim, *A Reporter's Own Story of AIDS in East Africa* (Bodley Head, 1990). Also of value is John Iliffe, *The African AIDS Epidemic: A History* (James Currey, 2006).

The original reports of the epidemic came from the *United States Centers for Disease Control Morbidity and Mortality Weekly Report* (5 June 1981).

Most of the data on the global epidemic is derived from the *UNAIDS Report on the Global Epidemic* (UNAIDS, 2006) and the UNAIDS website.

The South African data and Figure 1 come from Olive Shisana *et al.* (eds) *South African National HIV Prevalence, HIV Incidence, Behaviour and Communication Survey 2005* (HSRC Press, 2005).

The data on schools comes from *HIV Prevalence among South African Educators in Public Schools* (Human Sciences Research Council and Medical Research Council, 2005, Fact Sheet 6).

The information on the Nigerian army is from A. Adefalolu, 'HIV/AIDS as an Occupational Hazard to Soldiers – ECOMOG Experience', paper presented at the Third All Africa Congress of Armed Forces and Police Medical Services, Pretoria, South Africa, 1999. The Debswana data is from Barnett and Whiteside, and additional unpublished material.

Recent books include James Chin, *The AIDS Pandemic: The Collision of Epidemiology with Political Correctness* (Radcliffe Publishing, 2007), which argues that the scale of the epidemic in Asia was overstated, and Helen Epstein, *The Invisible Cure: Africa, the West, and the Fight against AIDS* (Farrow, Straus and Giroux, 2007), which seeks to understand the evolution of the epidemic in Africa.

Chapter 2

Trying to understand the virus is not undertaken lightly. Useful books are Barry D. Schoub, *AIDS and HIV in Perspective: A Guide to Understanding the Virus and its Consequences*, 2nd edn (Cambridge University Press, 1999); Michael B. A. Oldstone, *Viruses, Plagues and History* (Oxford University Press, 2000); and Jaap Goudsmit, *Viral Sex* (Oxford University Press, 1998).

The issue of HIV and TB is increasingly important. Of particular value are articles by Yan Wang, Charles Collins, Mercy Vergis, Nancy Gerein, and Jean Macq, 'HIV/AIDS and TB: Contextual Issues and Policy Choice in Programme Relations', *Tropical Medicine and International Health*, 12(2) (February 2007), and N. R. Gandhi *et al.*, 'Extensively Drug-Resistant Tuberculosis as a Cause of Death in Patients Co-Infected with Tuberculosis and HIV in a Rural Area of South Africa', *The Lancet*, 368 (9547) (November 2006).

The early work on circumcision was from John C. Caldwell *et al.* (eds) *Resistances to Behavioural Change to Reduce HIV/AIDS Infection* (Health Transition Centre, Australian National University, 1989). The most recent and most important document is from WHO and UNAIDS, *New Data on Male Circumcision and HIV Prevention: Policy and Programme Implications* (WHO/UNAIDS Technical Consultation, Male Circumcision and HIV Prevention: Research Implications for Policy and Programming, Montreux, 6–8 March 2007).

For information on vaccines, see www.iavi.org; for microbicides, see www.ipm-microbicides.org.

Chapter 3

The discussion of AIDS, nutrition, and poverty is excellently captured by Eileen Stillwaggon, *AIDS and the Ecology of Poverty* (Oxford University Press, 2006). The role of malaria was assessed by Laith J. Abu-Raddad, Padmaja Patnaik, and James G. Kublin, 'Dual Infection with HIV and Malaria Fuels the Spread of Both Diseases in Sub-Saharan Africa', *Science* (8 December 2006).

Interesting writing on sexual behaviours is taken from Soori Nnko, J. Ties Boerma, Mark Urassa, Gabriel Mwaluko, and Basia Zaba, *Secretive Females or Swaggering Males? An Assessment of the Quality of Sexual Partnership Reporting in Rural Tanzania* (Population Center, University of North Carolina at Chapel Hill, 2002), www.cpc.unc.edu/measure/publications/pdf/wp-02-57.pdf.

The only meta-analysis of sexual behaviour data comes from Kaye Wellings, Martine Collumbien, Emma Slaymaker, Susheela Singh, Zoé Hodges, Dhaval Patel, and Nathalie Bajos, 'Sexual Behaviour in Context: A Global Perspective', *The Lancet* (11 November 2006). Data are also drawn from the Durex Global Sex Survey, www.durex.com; the Demographic and Health Surveys, http://www.measuredhs.com/; and the Reproductive Health Research

Unit, HIV and Sexual Behaviour among Young South Africans, A National Survey of 15–24 Year Olds (2004), http://www.rhru.co.za/content/files/documents/National_Youth_Survey_Fact_Sheet.pdf.

The seminal article on concurrency of partnering is Daniel T. Halperin and Helen Epstein, 'Concurrent Sexual Partnerships Help to Explain Africa's High HIV Prevalence: Implications for Prevention', *The Lancet*, 364(9428) (3–9 July 2004): 4–6.

The model showing impact of focused intervention in Kenya is from the World Bank, *Confronting AIDS: Public Priorities in a Global Epidemic. A World Bank Policy Research Report* (Oxford University Press for the World Bank, European Commission, and UNAIDS, 1997).

An attempt to identify the drivers of the epidemic in Swaziland is Alan Whiteside, Catarina Andrade, Lisa Arrehag, Solomon Dlamini, Themba Ginindza, and Anokhi Parikh, *The Socio-Economic Impact of HIV/AIDS in Swaziland* (HIV AIDS Economic Research Division and NERCHA, 2006), on the HEARD website.

Chapter 4

Demographic data are drawn from the US Census Bureau, *The AIDS Pandemic in the 21st Century* (US Government Printing Office, 2004), International Population Reports WP/02-2 (2004), and United Nations Population Division, Department of Economic and Social Affairs, *The Impact of AIDS* (United Nations, 2004).

The South African data are from *Mortality and Causes of Death in South Africa, 1997–2003: Findings from Death Notification* (Statistics SA, February 2005).

The article on the effect of a mother's death was by Marie-Louse Newell, Heena Brahmbatt, and Peter H. Ghys, 'Child Mortality and HIV Infection in Africa', *AIDS*, 18(2) (June 2004).

The Actuarial Society of South Africa has data and models at www.assa.org.za.

Chapter 5

The impact of HIV/AIDS has been central to my research, see Tony Barnett and Alan Whiteside, *AIDS in the Twenty-First Century: Disease and Globalization*, 2nd edn (Palgrave, 2006). A useful framing publication is Hein Marais, *Buckling: The Impact of AIDS in South Africa, 2005* (Centre for the Study of AIDS, University of Pretoria, 2005).

The best empirical work on HIV/AIDS and its impact comes from the Center for International Health and Development at Boston University. Four papers need specific reference: Sydney Rosen, Rich Feeley, Patrick Connelly, and Jonathon Simon, 'The Private Sector and HIV/AIDS in Africa: Taking Stock of Six Years of Applied Research', Health and Development Discussion Paper No. 7 (June 2006); M. Fox, S. Rosen, W. MacLeod, M. Wasunna, M. Bii, G. Foglia, and J. Simon, 'The Impact of HIV/AIDS on Labour Productivity in Kenya', *Tropical Medicine and International Health*, 9 (2004): 318–24; Bruce Larson, Petan Hamazakaza, Crispin Kapunda, Coillard Hamusimbi, and Sydney Rosen, 'Morbidity, Mortality, and Crop Production: An Empirical Study of Smallholder Cotton Growing Households in the Central Province of Zambia' (2004); and Frank Feeley, Maggie Banda, Sydney Rosen, and Matthew Fox, 'The Impact of HIV/AIDS on the Judicial System in the Republic of Zambia' (2006) – all available from the Center for International Health and Development website http://sph.bu.edu/index. php?option=com_content&task=view&id=427&Itemid=526.

Priscilla's story is taken from Save the Children, *Missing Mothers: Meeting the Needs of Children Affected by AIDS* (Save the Children UK, 2006), p. 4.

In the discussion on AIDS and agriculture the 'new variant famine' ideas were published in Alex De Waal and Alan Whiteside, 'New Variant Famine: AIDS and Food Crisis in Southern Africa', *The Lancet*, 362 (9391) (11 October 2003): 1234–7. The Malawi data comes from Anne C. Conroy, Malcolm J. Blackie, Alan Whiteside, Justin C. Malewezi, and Jeffrey D. Sachs, *Poverty, AIDS and Hunger: Breaking the Poverty Trap in Malawi* (Palgrave, 2006), while those for Zimbabwe are from P. Kwaramba, 'The Socio-Economic Impact of HIV/AIDS on Communal Agricultural Production Systems in Zimbabwe' (Economic Advisory Project, Friedrich Ebert Stiftung, Harare, 1998, Working Paper 19), and the Famine Early Warning Network, www.fews.net.

The work on grandmothers and Warwick Junction is drawn from May Chazan's excellent ethnographic research presented at the International AIDS Conference in Toronto in 2006, 'What Will Happen When Grandmothers Die? Unpacking the Gender and Generational Implications of Aids and Household Changes among Street Traders in Durban, South Africa' (Abstract WEAD0101).

The role of health in development is from the WHO, *Macroeconomics and Health: Investing in Health for Economic Development* (Commission on Macroeconomics and Health, 2001).

Chapter 6

The politics of AIDS in South Africa is described by Pieter Fourie, *Political Management of HIV/AIDS in South Africa: One Burden too Many* (Palgrave, 2006) and Nicoli Nattrass, *Mortal Combat: AIDS Denialism and the Fight for Antiretrovirals in South Africa* (University of KwaZulu-Natal Press, 2007).

The links between AIDS and conflict were postulated by, among others, Martin Schönteich, 'Age and AIDS: South Africa's Crime Time Bomb', *AIDS Analysis Africa*, 10(2) (August/September 1999), and countered by Laurie Garrett, 'HIV and National Security: Where Are the Links?' (Council on Foreign Relations Report, 2005); Alan Whiteside, Alex De Waal, and Tsadkan Gebre-Tensae, 'AIDS, Security, and the Military in Africa: A Sober Appraisal', *African Affairs*, 105(419) (2006): 201–18; and Tony Barnett and Gwyn Prins, 'HIV/AIDS and Security: Fact, Fiction and Evidence, a Report to UNAIDS' (London School of Economics for UNAIDS, 2005).

The Zimbabwe hypothesis is by Andrew T. Price-Smith and John L. Daly, *Downward Spiral: HIV/AIDS, State Capacity, and Political Conflict in Zimbabwe* (United States Institute of Peace, 2004, Peaceworks No. 53).

The data from the Afrobarometer are available from www.afrobarometer.org. The original analysis is in Alan Whiteside, Robert Mattes, Samantha Willan, and Ryann Manning, 'Examining the HIV/AIDS Epidemic in Southern Africa Through the Eyes of Ordinary Southern Africans' (Afrobarometer, 2003, Working Paper No. 21). The analysis of the 2004 election in South Africa is by Per Strand and Kondwani Chirambo (eds), 'HIV/AIDS and Democratic Governance in South Africa: Illustrating the Impact on Electoral Process' (IDASA, 2004). Other and more recent publications are available on their website www.idasa.org.za

Data on international aid come from Jennifer Kates, J. Stephen Morrison, and Eric Lief, 'Funding for Global Health in Developing Countries by the United States and Europe, 2000–2004', paper prepared for Enhanced US-European Action to Strengthen the Governance of International Health (12–13 March 2006).

Chapter 7

The responses to the epidemic have been covered in a number of publications, in the mainstream were Jonathan Mann and Daniel Tarantola (eds), *AIDS in the World II* (Oxford University Press, 1996); Laurie Garrett, *The Coming Plague: Newly Emerging Diseases in a*

World Out of Balance (Penguin, 1995); and Laurie Garrett, *Betrayal of Trust: The Collapse of Global Public Health* (Hyperion, 2000).

Issues around sexuality are explored in Jared Diamond, *Why Is Sex Fun? The Evolution of Human Sexuality* (Weidenfeld and Nicolson, 1997), and applied to HIV/AIDS by Alex De Waal and Alan Whiteside, 'AIDS, a Darwinian Event', in Phillipe Denis and Charles Becker (eds), *The HIV/AIDS Epidemic in Sub-Saharan Africa in a Historical Perspective* (2006), http://www refer sn/rds/article php3?id_article=245.

Chapter 8

The parallels between AIDS and climate change are explored in May Chazan, M. Brklacich, and Alan Whiteside, 'Rethinking the Complexities of AIDS Impact: A Call for Interdisciplinarity', AIDS 2006 – XVI International AIDS Conference, 2006 (Abstract No. THAD0204).

The *Lancet* editorial appeared in July 2004: 'HIV/AIDS: Not One Epidemic But Many', *The Lancet*, 364(9428) (3 July 2004): 1–2.

The issues of economics and choice are explored in Sydney Rosen, Ian Sanne, Alizanne Collier, and Jonathon L. Simon, 'Rationing Antiretroviral Therapy for HIV/AIDS in Africa: Choices and Consequences', *Public Library of Science Medicine*, 2(11), e303, (November 2005): 1098; and by Sabrina Lee and Alan Whiteside, 'The "Free by 5" Campaign for Universal, Free Antiretroviral Therapy: User Fees Pose a Significant Barrier to Achievement of the "3 by 5" Strategy', *Public Library of Science Medicine*, 2(8) (August 2005). On the human resource question, see Debbie Palmer, 'Tackling Malawi's Human Resources Crisis', *Reproductive Health Matters*, 14(27) (2006): 27–39; and Gorik Ooms, Wim Van Damme, and Marleen Temmerman, 'Medicines without Doctors: Why the Global Fund Must Fund Salaries of Health Workers to Expand AIDS Treatment', *Public Library of Science Medicine*, 4(4) (April 2007).

Index

Visit the
VERY SHORT
INTRODUCTIONS
Web site

www.oup.co.uk/vsi

➤ **Information** about all published titles

➤ News of **forthcoming books**

➤ **Extracts** from the books, including titles not yet published

➤ **Reviews** and views

➤ **Links** to other **web sites** and main OUP web page

➤ Information about **VSIs in translation**

➤ **Contact** the editors

➤ **Order** other **VSIs** on-line